CPAP and
SECRETS

LIVE, BREATHE & SLEEP
WITH NON-INVASIVE VENTILATION

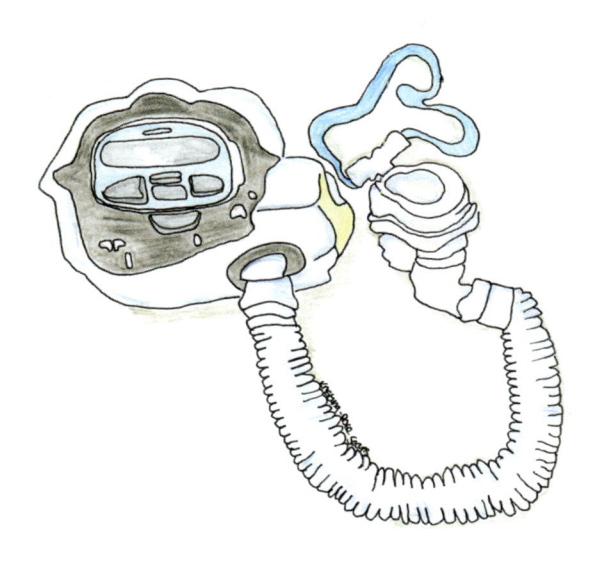

Marion Maz Mason with Steve B. Mason

Foreword by
Dr J M Shneerson MA DM FRCP

Artwork by Kristina-Rose Sears

As I Live and Breathe

Copyright © 2011 Marion Maz Mason & Steve B Mason

Artwork copyright © 2011 Kristina-Rose Sears

All rights reserved.

The right of Marion Maz Mason and Steve B Mason to be identified as the authors of this work has been asserted in accordance with the Copyright, Designs and Patents Act 1988.

No portion of this book may be reproduced, in whole or in part, or transmitted in any form, electronic or mechanical including photocopying, recording and information storage and retrieval, without the prior written permission of the publisher, nor be otherwise circulated in any form of binding or cover other than that in which it is published and without similar conditions being imposed on the subsequent publisher.

British Library Cataloguing in Publication Data
A catalogue record for this book is available from The British Library

Published by
As I Live and Breathe
www.asiliveandbreathe.co.uk

ISBN 978-0-9569455-1-8

Printed by Gipping Press
Needham Market U.K.

DISCLAIMER

Information in this book is provided for informational and entertainment purposes only and is not meant to substitute the advice provided by your own physician or other medical professional. You should not use the information contained herein for diagnosing or treating a health problem or disease, or prescribing any medication.

Use the information at your own risk. No guarantee is made towards validity.

You should read all equipment manuals and instructions carefully.

If you have or suspect that you have a medical problem, promptly contact your health care provider. You should not discontinue or modify any medication or treatment presently being taken under medical advice without first obtaining approval from your healthcare professional.

Information and statements regarding dietary supplements, medicines, exercises, conditions, illnesses, treatments and therapies, have not been evaluated by any medical practitioner, agency, or governing body, and are not intended to diagnose, treat, cure, or prevent any virus, disease or condition.

The authors and publisher shall not accept liability or responsibility to any person with respect to loss, injury or damage caused or alleged to be caused by information within this book.

About the authors

Marion Mason

Marion is an experienced tutor in Adult Education, specialising in whole-food and vegetarian cooking. She is actively involved with The Scoliosis Association UK and other organisations for people with disabilities.

Born with congenital scoliosis, she developed severe respiratory problems in later life. Thanks to mechanical ventilation support at night-time, she continues to lead a full and productive life.

This book is the result of her experience and research.

Steve Mason

Marion's son Steve has extensive experience of NIV from observing and caring for his mother. He has gained further knowledge from his father who uses CPAP therapy for Sleep Apnoea.

He is a Reiki Master, and has studied Traditional Chinese Medicine, as well as Complementary Therapies including Massage, Hypnotherapy and NLP (Neuro-Linguistic Programming).

CONTENTS

FOREWORD
By Dr J M Shneerson MA DM FRCP

ACKNOWLEDGEMENTS

EARLY DAYS

Part 1
INTRODUCTION

ABOUT THIS BOOK	1
HOW THIS BOOK CAN HELP YOU	3

CHAPTER 1   5
WHAT IS NON-INVASIVE VENTILATION?
  What is NIV?
  Who uses it?
  What is a sleep study?

Part 2
TAKING CARE OF PRACTICALITIES & PROBLEMS

CHAPTER 2   17
CARE OF YOUR EQUIPMENT
  How should I set up my CPAP / ventilator?
  I have a humidifier unit
  How can I tell if the machine is faulty?
  How should I clean my machine?
  I think my device contains replaceable filters.
  How do I clean my mask?
  What about the hose?
  Should I wash my headgear & chin-strap in the washing machine?

CHAPTER 3   25
USING THE EQUIPMENT
How can I call to my family if I need them during the night?
How do I choose the right mask for me?
I'm new to this and am having a problem positioning the straps.
How can I stop air leaks?
When I am lying on my side my mask gets pushed up by my pillow.
My teeth hurt in the morning!
I have a moustache: will it get in the way of my mask?
My arm gets caught up in the hose while I'm asleep.
My mouth doesn't stay closed while I sleep.
My throat gets sore at night.
My nose gets cold.
The straps leave marks on my cheeks.
What should I do if there's a power cut in the night?

CHAPTER 4   37
SKINCARE
I'm a man – surely I needn't bother with skincare?
How can I prevent the mask making my face sore?
Can I use ordinary soap on my face?
What about moisturising?
Should I stay out of the sun?
I am embarrassed by the red patches on my face.
My face is very sore.
Would vitamin supplements help my skin?

CHAPTER 5   45
GENERAL HEALTH ISSUES
How can I deal with a blocked nose?
I've been suffering from bloating.
What about alcohol? I like to have a drink with my mates.
My G.P. doesn't know much about my condition.
My doctor doesn't understand the difference between CPAP & my ventilator.
Some medical personnel don't seem to understand my condition.
Would I have difficulties during surgery?
I am sensitive to household chemicals & perfumes.
What else could have an effect on my breathing?
My toenails have changed. Could my condition be to blame?

CHAPTER 6   57
TRAVEL
- Anything else I should take with my ventilator?
- My condition got worse when I went to Aviemore in Scotland
- Should I ask my Doctor about air travel?
- Will I be able to get travel insurance?
- Do I need to carry a letter from my Doctor?
- Hand luggage or baggage hold?

Part 3
TAKING CARE OF RELATIONSHIPS & FEELINGS

CHAPTER 7   65
YOUR EMOTIONS & YOU
- It's all a bit daunting at the moment.
- Friends have noticed my low self-esteem.
- I can't do all the things I used to.
- I think I'll try a new hobby now.
- I don't like being dependent on a machine.
- Where else can I get advice & support?

CHAPTER 8   73
FAMILY, FRIENDS & WORK
- I don't want to scare my children.
- My family is taking it harder than me!
- It's hard to make my friends understand.
- I'd like to carry on at my job.
- I'd like to meet people and make new friends who understand my situation.

CHAPTER 9   81
DATING & RELATIONSHIPS
- I want to start dating again but have lost confidence and feel unattractive.
- How do I tell my new partner about it?
- I'm afraid my partner will be horrified.
- Won't the noise keep my partner awake?

What about our intimate moments?
As a woman I do feel unattractive now.

CHAPTER 10 — 101
DEALING WITH THE FEELINGS
The 'Arrow' Method:
A Self-Help Technique for dealing with anxiety & negative emotions.

Part 4
TAKING CARE OF YOURSELF

CHAPTER 11 — 111
SENSITIVITY TO INDOOR POLLUTION
    General advice
    Bathroom
    Bedroom
    Air Freshener products
    Laundry
    Tobacco and smoke
    Pets
    Wooden & vinyl floors

CHAPTER 12 — 117
HEALTH INFORMATION FOR EMERGENCIES
    Should I carry health information in case of a medical emergency?
    Medic-Alert
    SOS-Talisman
    The Lions Club 'Message in a Bottle' scheme
    The I.C.E. system

CHAPTER 13 — 123
DIET & NUTRITION
    Should I see my Doctor about my weight?
    I've tried lots of celebrity diets but they don't work
    I couldn't possibly give up chocolate
    I don't eat unless I'm really hungry
    I just can't face food first thing in the morning
    I often feel peckish

What are the tips for a 'Diet for Life'?
> Cutting down on snacks
> Meal times
> Eating out

It's hard to do it alone
I weigh myself daily to see how much I've lost
Is home-cooking worth the effort?
Sometimes I'm too tired or unwell to cook a proper meal
My problem is that I'm underweight

CHAPTER 14 — 135
SMOKING
Will it really make a difference if I give up smoking?
What's the best way of giving up?
How can I kick the habit?
I need help to give up cigarettes.
What else can I do to help myself?
Will I put on weight if I stop smoking?

CHAPTER 15 — 141
EXERCISE
My breathing problems make exercise difficult
At the Gym – For the more active person
Won't I get fat if I stop exercising?
Exercising would quickly bore me.
Exercise ideas, including sitting exercises
> Resistance Bands
> Weights
> P.T. Exercises – Callisthenics
> Dancing
> Yoga
> Tai Chi
> Pilates
> Singing

I'd like to go swimming.
I like the water but can't manage to swim.

Part 5
PRESENT DAY   153

APPENDICES   157

Appendix I   GLOSSARY OF TERMS AND ACRONYMS
Appendix II   CONTACTS LIST

INDEX

FOREWORD

More and more people are now using mechanical equipment to help with their difficulties in breathing during sleep. This is usually a continuous positive pressure (CPAP) system for sleep apnoeas but others need more sophisticated equipment in the form of a ventilator. This can be disconcerting and raises questions and concerns about a large number of issues. Up until now it has been hard to find the answers to these, but this book fills this gap. It is written specifically for the CPAP and ventilator user and highlights common issues that arise.

The book takes a wide ranging approach, including information not only on the mechanics of the equipment and how to look after it, but also how to use both CPAP and ventilators in a way which enables the user to make the most of their life. Problems that arise are identified clearly and it is easy to find the way through the chapters. The emphasis is on the need to make the equipment not only resolve problems with breathing and sleep but also to fit it into the everyday lifestyle issues that people face. There will hardly be any CPAP or ventilator user who will not learn a lot from this book and be able to manage their condition, their equipment and their life better.

Dr J M Shneerson MA DM FRCP
Consultant Physician
Respiratory Support and Sleep Centre
Papworth Hospital
Papworth Everard
Cambridge
U.K.

ACKNOWLEDGEMENTS

With thanks to:-

Dr John Shneerson, for believing in the book, and for kindly providing a foreword

Steve Mason, for adapting portions of his Arrow Method for this book

All my research participants and contributors. Your stories moved me and inspired me to write this book. This is for you!

Dr Jonathan Douse, for his interest and encouragement

Elizabeth Gwilliam, for inspiration, encouragement and proof-reading skills

Giles Meehan, for editorial input

Wendy Guevara, whose album provided musical motivation when writing seemed an impossible task

Kristina-Rose Sears, for her artwork

Photographic model Steve Whiting

J Bilner for CPAP photographs

EARLY DAYS

When they brought the machine to me, and said I would always need it, I was appalled.

"I'll never cope with having this thing over my face," I thought, *"and it's Goodbye to ever leading a normal life again."*

I was wrong on both counts.

Marion M Mason

Part 1
INTRODUCTION

About This Book

I am not aware of any other book which would provide so much helpful information to people who need ventilatory support.

Dr J Shneerson, Papworth Hospital

This easy-to-read book addresses queries and problems arising from the use of Non-Invasive Ventilation (NIV) equipment at home. It is a practical guide to many common difficulties experienced by users of this kind of therapy.

The book aims to bridge the gap between the initial information given on discharge from hospital, and the various problems which the user may encounter at home. It aims to reduce common anxieties and the sense of isolation felt by some people who live with NIV. In addition it aims to help increase their confidence in the therapy, encouraging them to take an active part in their own health care.

As well as information on setting up and using the equipment, the book covers general health questions, smoking, exercise, diet & nutrition, family, relationships and dealing with anxiety or negative emotions. Some of these chapters will be of interest to people who have other medical problems, and perhaps even to those with no disability at all. Nursing staff, family members, and support groups may also benefit from reading this book.

NIV is prescribed to treat many different conditions, and various types of ventilator and equipment are used for such therapies. We use terms such as equipment, ventilator and machine to refer to the NIV equipment in general terms.

This book covers issues and problems that are common to many NIV users, while other topics covered may be relevant to fewer people, depending on their own personal circumstances. Included is a list of useful contacts, support groups and telephone help lines.

Marion Mason (author) has over twenty years personal experience of using mechanically-assisted ventilation, and this book includes contributions and anecdotes from users of NIV who participated in her research project.

The information and advice offered in this book is not intended as a substitute for professional medical advice.
It represents information and points of view gathered from the real-life experiences of the author and her research participants.

1

How This Book Can Help You

Thinking back, it would have been very useful to have a book like this. We had nothing, and at first you struggle in the dark – literally!

Carer of NIV patient

It can be quite a daunting prospect, when you first arrive home with this piece of medical equipment that will help you to breathe, but the hospital medical staff did a grand job – they showed you how to put on the mask, and switch on the machine, explained how often you should use it, gave you a date for your follow-up appointment, and assured you that you will feel much better from now on.

You follow their instructions, and get on with managing your health at home as best you can. All goes well until, one day, a query or problem arises about which you'd like some advice –

Plan A - Check the machine's User Guide Manual

You turn to the manual they gave you with the equipment: it's a thick booklet, in seven languages, full of system specifications, electromagnetic emissions, manufacturer's declarations, and other scientific jargon! It includes some basic user instructions, but its technical info is of little use for your query.

Plan B – Ask somebody

If it's a medical issue, of course you should contact your G.P. or Consultant for advice; but maybe you are reluctant to bother your busy doctor or hospital unit with what seems like a trivial non-medical matter.

So who can you ask? Where can you get support? Who will understand? Typically you would prefer to turn to other people who are in a similar situation to yourself, and who have perhaps had longer experience of it. Or could you ask your family, friends, or a Pharmacist?

Various factors can make these options difficult:-

- Maybe it's too embarrassing to discuss with friends and family
- You fear that people will not understand that something which sounds quite minor to them can have greater implications for you
- You wonder whether they will think you are exaggerating the problem for sympathy
- They don't know anything about the subject anyway!
- You don't know anyone with a similar condition
- You are not aware of a relevant support group that you could contact

This book has been written to try to provide help for you. Hopefully within its pages you will find the information you need, plus links to useful organisations and websites.

Never delay in seeking individual advice from your Doctor because of something you have read in this book.

CHAPTER 1

What is Non-Invasive Ventilation (NIV)?

I've been on NIV since the 1980s. In those days my hospital was still using Iron Lungs which they had salvaged from other hospitals, but I had a Cuirass at first, then a Monnal D. This was later replaced by a Nippy, followed by a BIPAP, which I am using now.

BIPAP user

What is NIV?
Mechanical ventilation equipment

Non-Invasive Ventilation, or NIV, is the provision of ventilatory support through a patient's upper airway, using a mask or other similar device. Air under pressure is delivered to the patient by means of a small machine, or ventilator.

If you've ever taken first-aid classes you will have learned about mouth-to-mouth resuscitation, also known as The Kiss of Life. This simple form of non-mechanical ventilation has often saved lives in emergency situations. There have been reports, dating back many years, of its use in reviving asphyxiated or drowning people, and in helping newborn babies to commence breathing.

But a more efficient way of assisting people to breathe was needed for those undergoing surgery. Advances were made in developing mechanical methods, especially when complicated and lengthy surgical procedures became possible. Artificial ventilators were introduced into the anaesthetic process during operations, using invasive methods such as a tracheostomy - an opening that is made in the front of the trachea or windpipe, through which to ventilate the patient.

As well as developing ventilation machines for use during surgical operations, there was research into other types of equipment for treating long-term lung patients. They needed non-invasive methods of ventilation, and 'negative pressure ventilators' were produced for this purpose.

A **negative pressure ventilator:** takes control of the patient's breathing actions. It works by enclosing the patient's body inside a tank or jacket, and reducing the air pressure inside. This causes the patient's lungs to expand, and air is drawn into their lungs through their mouth. The pressure is then returned to normal. The patient exhales passively because of the elastic recoil of the chest wall and the lungs.

The Iron Lung is a tank respirator, a large, bulky and rigid negative pressure chamber, in which the patient lies enclosed from the neck downwards. These Iron Lungs had been used since the late 1920s for long-term respiratory care associated with conditions such as Polio. However, epidemics of the disease during the 1950s hastened research into mechanical respiratory support, as smaller and more portable equipment was urgently needed for the large number of Polio patients requiring ventilators.

Equipment that was more compact, such as the Cuirass, was developed. The Cuirass is a negative pressure chamber, or shell, which is smaller than an Iron Lung but performs a similar function and can be used in a domestic situation. It encloses only the patient's thorax – the part of the body enclosed by the rib cage - and is connected by a large hose to pumping equipment beside the patient's bed. It is made from a material such as fibreglass and, for best results, is individually made from a cast of the patient's body.

Jacket ventilators have also been used, consisting of an air-tight garment which seals around the arms, waist and neck and is held rigid by an inner framework. It is connected to a pump in the same manner as a cuirass.

Positive Pressure ventilators: work by increasing the pressure within the airways. This is achieved by delivering compressed air to the patient's nose, via a mask. Unlike tank respirators, these machines do not take control of the patient's breathing, although some can do so should the patient fail to breathe spontaneously.

Developments in positive airway pressure ventilators have resulted in equipment that a patient can use conveniently at home, thus avoiding a prolonged hospital stay. An early model of a portable ventilator is the Monnal D. About the size of a medium suitcase, it is transportable but heavy.

Smaller machines, for example the Non-Invasive Positive Pressure Ventilator (NIPPY) and Bi-Level Positive Airways Pressure Ventilator (BIPAP), have now taken over from the likes of the Monnal D and the Cuirass. Continuous Positive Airway Pressure (CPAP) machines are used to treat patients with Sleep Apnoea.

Modern ventilators are smaller and lighter than previous versions. The moving parts which perform the pneumatic pumping action are more compact and are situated internally, and the bulk of the machine consists of an electronic unit.

> *My Monnal D performed its job brilliantly, but it was so heavy – it took both my husband and my son to lift it! But it didn't stop us going away on holiday. We always travelled with a local coach company that handled my machine with great care. Now I have a Nippy ventilator and it's so much easier. I can lift it by myself, and pop it into the boot of my car.*

Research continues, and updated equipment is brought into use. There is now a CPAP machine small enough to fit into the palm of your hand, and the NIPPY3, with its colour LCD display screen, replaces the larger, heavier NIPPY1 & 2.

Who uses NIV?
How does it help them with their breathing difficulties during sleep?

Several different conditions can lead to respiratory difficulties, and a variety of NIV ventilators are used in their treatment.

Sleep Apnoea and CPAP ventilators

Perhaps the most well-known condition that can benefit from mechanically assisted ventilation therapy is Obstructive Sleep Apnoea (OSA), often associated with chronic snoring. With Sleep Apnoea a person's air passageways collapse during sleep, restricting the amount of air getting through. This difficulty in breathing causes them to snore and continually wake up gasping for breath, usually many times during the night. It leads to lowered levels of oxygen in the blood and extreme day-time tiredness.

Snoring has often been the subject of jokes, but it's no laughing matter. It can, in fact, indicate the potentially dangerous condition of OSA, with its associated risks of raised blood pressure, stroke and heart attack.

Sleep Apnoea can have several causes, but is often a problem for the overweight and obese. Its incidence is rising with the trend towards heavier body weight and obesity among the general population. Anyone who suspects that they have this condition should seek medical advice, as OSA could have serious consequences if not treated.

Continual sleep-deprivation caused by sleep disturbance every night can have a major impact on health, both physically and emotionally. It leads to severe day-time drowsiness, exhaustion, memory lapses, fatigue and lack of concentration. This is especially dangerous for vehicle drivers or machinery operators. It can be a contributory factor in road traffic accidents and industrial injuries. People's jobs can be affected, and the driving licence of a person with OSA may be withdrawn if they are not having medical treatment for the condition.

Also, of course, when someone in the family snores heavily there is a knock-on effect for other family members. They also suffer from noisy, disturbed nights and lack of sleep, while the snorer and their partner may develop relationship problems, sometimes resulting in an increased risk of divorce!

A Continuous Positive Airways Pressure (CPAP) machine is used in the treatment of OSA, for patients who are able to breathe spontaneously. The patient wears a close-fitting mask covering the nose, or a slightly larger mask covering the nose and the mouth. This is held in place by straps around the back of the head, above and below the ears, and is connected by a hose to the bedside CPAP machine. The CPAP gently and quietly pumps ambient air, under pressure, via a flow generator through the hose and into the mask. This provides a continuous pressurised air supply through the nose. The pressure of this air gently inflates the throat and holds open the relaxed muscles of the patient's airways during sleep. It prevents the airways from collapsing, and allows the patient to breathe normally.

The CPAP machine provides a highly effective home treatment for OSA and, being small and easily portable, it is light enough to take away on holidays. It enables the user to breathe naturally while asleep, and improves the quality of that sleep. Blood oxygen levels are maintained, snoring and daytime sleepiness are reduced or eliminated, and the patient no longer feels permanently exhausted. The CPAP brings welcome relief to the snorer and to the family.

Bi-level and Nippy Positive Pressure Ventilators

Some people with skeletal deformity or weak respiratory muscles have restricted lung capacities or inefficient respiration, which makes breathing spontaneously when asleep particularly problematic. Because of their depressed breathing these people find it difficult to take in sufficient oxygen and to eliminate excess carbon dioxide from the body. In some cases the automatic breathing reflex is impaired. For patients like these mechanical ventilation is required every time they sleep. They do not use a CPAP, but require a different type of machine – a ventilator such as a Non-Invasive Positive Pressure Ventilator (NIPPV - often referred to as a Nippy).

Instead of the continuous air flow of a CPAP, a Nippy ventilator gives pulses of air under pressure, which expand and fill the lungs. These bursts of air are coupled with a few seconds when there is low air input, or none at all. As a result, this period of low pressure enables the sleeper's lungs to deflate and expel the air. This cycle replicates the normal process of breathing in and out, and helps the patient by topping up the volume of air that they inhale. The machine is triggered by the user's own efforts to take a breath, but the machine can also initiate a breath if the patient himself fails to breathe spontaneously within a pre-set period of time. The machine's assistance also helps to relieve the respiratory muscles by reducing the effort needed to breathe.

Bi-level Positive Airways Pressure (BIPAP or Bi-PAP) ventilators work in a similar way; they have two levels of pressure – the inspiratory pressure (when the patient breathes in) and a lower expiratory pressure (when the patient breathes out). The NIPPY3 uses two levels of pressure. Other ventilators include the VPAP and BREAS.

Mechanically assisted ventilation therapy may be helpful for a wide variety of conditions including Scoliosis, Post-Polio Syndrome, neuromuscular disorders, Motor Neurone Disease, Parkinson's, Muscular Dystrophy, brainstem damage, and OSA that is unresponsive to CPAP. Recent research appears to show that patients with mild heart failure may also benefit from mechanical respiratory support.

Some patients may need NIV for part of the waking day, as well as during sleep, or may require additional oxygen sometimes.

What is a Sleep Study?

Sleep studies are conducted in order to assist the diagnosis of breathing disorders. Signs of such a problem developing can include: disturbed sleep, gasping and snoring during sleep, waking from sleep feeling breathless or panicky, morning headaches, daytime drowsiness, difficulty concentrating, and increasing breathlessness on exertion. Other conditions - Myalgic Encephalitis (ME) and depression, for example - can sometimes bring on similar symptoms, so a Sleep Study will help give a clearer picture of the patient's health.

Results from the tests will indicate the extent of the patient's respiratory condition, whether treatment is required, and which kind of treatment would be most suitable. Because some breathing conditions develop slowly, and may not require treatment for some time, the patient may be asked to undergo a Sleep Study on a regular basis – perhaps annually – so that monitoring of their health can continue.

During a Sleep Study many things can be measured without the use of needles or invasive devices.

> *I had an overnight stay in hospital because I changed from a Nippy ventilator to a BREAS and the settings on the new machine needed to be assessed. My blood gases were tested every few hours during the night. It didn't bother me, and proved worthwhile as they had to make significant adjustments to the settings. Periodically the hospital sends me an oximeter through the post, in order for me to do a sleep test at home – I return the equipment by post.*

A simple Oximetry test can measure and record blood oxygen levels and heart rate during sleep. This test can sometimes be done at home, and may not involve an overnight stay in hospital. A small device called an oximeter is used. It is strapped around the wrist like a wristwatch and has a sensor which is worn on one finger. Information on blood oxygen levels and heart-rate is recorded and the data stored on a memory chip. This data can then be downloaded for computer analysis when the gadget is returned to the Sleep Study Centre.

An overnight study in the hospital Sleep Study Centre can involve tests of a more involved nature. There may be lung function tests to check your lung capacity and the action of your breathing muscles, and a blood sample is sometimes taken. To measure your heart-rate and blood gases levels there are various simple overnight tests.

You will go to bed as usual, possibly in a private room. During the night blood oxygen levels can be monitored by the use of a pulse oximeter. This resembles a small plastic peg and is clipped onto a finger. It shines a light through the soft tissues of your finger, and painlessly measures the level of oxygen in your blood. It is hardly noticeable and shouldn't disturb you, although if you prefer you could ask for it to be attached to your ear or a toe instead.

A sensor taped to the arm measures carbon dioxide levels. Sometimes a small sensor is placed under the nose to monitor airflow.

> *I was quite young when I had my first overnight Sleep Study. I remember I had pads stuck to me with masking tape and an oxygen monitor clipped onto my finger. My next Sleep Study was in the adult ward of the hospital. As before, I had to stay the night, and had the oxygen monitor on my finger. During the night it had to be moved from finger to finger because my fingers went numb, and I ended up with it on my toe! All the time I was having the study the machine that was checking my heart-rate beeped every two minutes, but it wasn't a problem.*

Some procedures involve an overnight stay in a 'Sleep Laboratory' room. This sounds impressive, but it's really just a private room with more gadgets! It isn't anything to be worried about. In a Sleep Lab room a video recording can be made during the night (under infra-red light) to identify periods of restlessness, wakefulness, and abnormal sleep. Occasionally tests of a more intricate nature may be used involving sensors on your body linked to computer equipment.

> *I once had an overnight test called Polysomnography. It involved having little electrode sensors all over my head, with some bands around my chest to detect breathing movements, as well as the usual peg on my finger for*

checking oxygen levels. It wasn't uncomfortable and I slept very well, but the sensors on my head took ages to attach. There were two doctors sticking them onto my scalp with some kind of glue, trying not to get my hair sticky. I guess it must have taken them at least an hour or more, and all the while they were chatting away about holidays and cars - it was just like being at the hairdressers!

Once your test results have been analysed the medical team will have a better understanding of your condition and how to proceed. Perhaps you'll be asked to return for a further Sleep Study in a few months, or you may be offered physiotherapy, medication or other treatments, as appropriate.

If it's decided that you do need mechanical support for your breathing, arrangements will be made to issue you with NIV equipment. The settings for pressure and air-flow etc. on your machine will be determined by your Sleep Study results.

You'll probably be brought back after a few weeks, to follow-up on your progress and ensure you are getting on well and feel comfortable with the air pressure, mask and fittings.

Don't assume that you must be very poorly if you've been put onto NIV – your Physician aims to introduce you to this form of treatment *before* your sleeping problems become severe enough to start interfering with your day-time functioning.

In Brief

- ◆ Mechanical Respiratory Support is used for breathing disorders arising from various medical conditions
- ◆ There are several forms of Non-Invasive Ventilation equipment suitable for home use
- ◆ Most sleep study tests are simple and do not always involve an overnight stay at the hospital
- ◆ Analysis of your Sleep Study results will help with the diagnosis of your condition and the prescription of suitable treatments

- Regular Sleep Studies and other tests are used in order to monitor your health and to gauge your progress
- Snoring, or other symptoms of breathing problems during sleep, should be reported to your Doctor, who will be able to arrange any necessary medical investigations

Part 2
TAKING CARE OF PRACTICALITIES & PROBLEMS

CHAPTER 2

Care of Your Equipment

Cleaning your respiratory equipment is essential to the life of the equipment and to your health.

CPAP Station

When non-invasive ventilation (NIV) equipment is issued to you, you will receive instructions on its use and maintenance. Once you get back home it's a good idea to take time to look through the User's Manual, which you should keep somewhere handy for reference. Then if any queries arise, or you can't remember what you were told at the hospital, you can refer to the manual for assistance.

This book will also help you with some of the questions that may arise, but if you are not able to find the answer to your query, or there's something you still don't understand about using or looking after your equipment, do contact your Specialist Unit for clarification and assistance.

Because of time constraints at the hospital I had only one hour of instruction as an out-patient, instead of the usual three. It took time for me to get used to it, and I'm sure it would have been easier if I'd had the full three hours.

Happily, the machine itself doesn't need a lot of looking after. Just check it over regularly, to ensure that dust hasn't accumulated on it. At the same time make sure that the machine, tubing, mask, filters, power cable and plug are all in good, undamaged condition.

If you or your partner feels concerned that the noise of your machine may disturb the night's sleep see **Chapter 9 Dating & Relationships** which includes some useful advice for dealing with this.

How should I set up my CPAP / Ventilator?

Set up your machine by your bed, close to an electric power point. Make sure to allow space all round for air to circulate, and do not place anything on top. Ensure it's not in a position where it could get knocked, or where someone could trip over the power cable. Don't leave long lengths of hose at the top of your bed, as these could twist around your head while you are asleep. The tubing should be able to move freely if you change position in your sleep.

Always take care when moving or transporting your equipment. If you are travelling, ensure it doesn't get mistreated on the journey, and make sure it is in a weather-proof bag or cover, to protect it from damp and moisture.

I have a humidifier unit

A humidifier is a piece of equipment used with a ventilator to help relieve soreness, sensitivity or dryness of the throat and nasal passages. See **Chapter 3 Using the Equipment**

When setting up your humidifier unit, refer to its user manual for the ideal position. There is a small reservoir of water inside the humidifier. Make sure to place the humidifier in a position where it cannot accidentally be knocked, in case water from the reservoir gets into your other equipment. To prevent any risk of this, the humidifier should be positioned lower than your CPAP or ventilator.

I am careful not to jog my humidifier, and it's positioned away from my ventilator.

Using a heated humidifier in a cool bedroom can cause moisture to condense in the hose. Droplets of water are formed, and these could drip down the tubing into the mask.

To help prevent this 'rain-out', try positioning your equipment at a level lower than your sleeping position, perhaps on a small table or shelf, so that your hose rises vertically up to bed level. This helps prevent the water drops from making their way along the tubing to your face. Or use a Hose-Lift as described in **Chapter 3 Using the Equipment**.

Raising the bedroom temperature would be helpful, as less condensation will form when the air temperature is warmer. For the same reason, you may need to adjust the humidifier's settings if your bedroom temperature drops in cold weather. Again, check the manual or get advice from your equipment supplier. Consider turning up the night-time setting on your bedroom's heating thermostat. There is also a smaller chance of condensation forming if you insulate the hose by wrapping it with bubble-wrap or fleecy fabric. You may prefer to purchase a purpose-made cover called a Tube Wrap, which can be easily secured in place around the hose. For suppliers see **Appendix II Contacts List**.

Using a Tube Wrap, or some other form of insulation, can also prove useful if you find that your nose gets very cold at night. As air makes its way through the long hose, its temperature can drop, but with the wrap in place, it may not drop so much, and your nose is less likely to get chilled.

If condensation does form overnight, hang up your tubing in the morning, allowing it to drain and dry out completely before reconnecting it.

The water in your humidifier will need to be regularly emptied and the water reservoir wiped dry, to prevent a build-up of mineral deposits and growth of moulds or bacteria.

How can I tell if the machine is faulty?

Modern ventilatory equipment is reliable and unlikely to develop faults, so there is no need to be unduly worried about this. Any potential problems will be spotted by the engineer when the machine has its regular service.

If faults do develop at home they are usually obvious, once you become familiar with using your machine. For example, you could notice that the equipment is making an unusual sound or the filters get dirty very quickly. Perhaps the settings have been accidentally changed and the pressure feels wrong, or you spot signs of wear and tear.

There is usually an alarm on these machines. The alarm will sound if there's a problem, like a power failure when you are using the machine, or your hose slipping off its connection.

The alarm on my new Nippy ventilator sometimes went off while I was asleep. It was very brief, but enough to wake me up and disturb my night's sleep. Eventually I decided to phone the hospital, and they realised that one of the pressure settings on the Nippy was too low, causing the alarm to go off needlessly. I was able to make the

> *adjustments myself, while they gave me instructions over the phone, and I had no further problems.*

Contact your hospital unit or supplier if you feel there is a problem. If the staff cannot sort it out over the phone, they will organise replacements.

> *I had a problem when I first went home with my Nippy ventilator. I noticed I couldn't breathe deeply enough before the next breath was initiated by the machine. As I was new to NIV I didn't know what was happening. I thought it was my fault, and it didn't occur to me to call the hospital for advice. However, within a couple of weeks I was back at the hospital for my follow-up Sleep Study, where they noticed the problem and adjusted the Nippy's settings to rectify it.*

How should I clean my machine?

Don't use any solvents or abrasives. Just keep it dust-free, and wipe off any marks with a cloth. Stubborn marks can be wiped off with a damp cloth, but always disconnect the power supply first.

I think my device contains replaceable filters

Some machines have washable filters, while other models have replaceable filters which have to be changed from time to time.

> *My Nippy has replaceable filters, and I know how to change them and where to get replacements. The outside filter is easy to change although the one inside is a bit fiddly.*

Read your user's manual, or ask your hospital unit for instructions. Filters can vary, depending on the model of machine. Some ventilators have two filters. There may be a square filter, made of thick gauze, positioned where the air is drawn into the machine, and a round plastic filter where the hose is attached to the equipment.

     You should check filters weekly for dirt or holes, and clean them or fit new ones as appropriate, when necessary. It's useful to have spare filters at home, so try to organise a small supply in case you should need them.

> *I was chatting to another patient when I was at the hospital, and I noticed that the external filter on her Nippy machine was very dirty. I recommended that she ask for a new one straight away. She didn't realise that the filters needed to be changed and had never checked them.*

It's difficult to say how often your filters will need to be changed. Timing will vary according to the type of equipment, the hours of use, and the quality of the air which is drawn into the filter. Regular checks are therefore important; a weekly examination is recommended. Why not check the filters at the same time as you change the bed linen? Making it part of the bed-changing routine will help you remember to do it.

Please note that you will need to replace the filters much more frequently if your machine is used in a dusty or smoky environment. See **Chapter 11 Sensitivity to Indoor Pollution**.

How do I clean my mask?

It's important to keep the mask clean. Facial oils, germs and secretions can accumulate on the mask causing damage to your skin, as well as weakening the mask itself. Before putting on your mask, make sure there is no skin cream on your face where the mask will sit.

Regular cleaning of the mask will help extend its life by preventing this build-up. See also **Chapter 4 Skin Care**. Give your mask a gentle, daily wipe with a damp cloth; do not rub it. Once a week, or as needed, swish it in a weak solution of warm water and mild shampoo or dish detergent. Do not use hot water as this can harden or perish the plastic.

Rinse and wipe the mask, then let it dry out, but don't leave it in direct sunlight. Make sure it is completely dry before re-connecting to your hose. Pay extra attention to cleaning it when you have a cold, cough or other infection, in order to keep it free of bacteria.

Don't be tempted to use household cleaning products on your mask - these are too harsh. Avoid using any product which contains alcohol, conditioners, perfumes or moisturisers as these will leave behind a residue. Do not use bleach. Cleansing Wipes and Sprays specially formulated for your equipment are available, though not essential. See **Appendix II Contacts List** for Equipment & Product Supplies.

Make sure that your mask is not fastened too tightly during use as this can make your skin sore. It increases wear on the straps and could damage the mask itself.

> *I have a mask which has a soft, blue cushion around it containing gel. It's very comfortable on my face and I get on with it very well. I do wipe it clean every day and check it, because the plastic cushion can eventually break down through wear and tear, especially if the mask is on too tight. It's happened once: one night my mask split while I was asleep and I woke with something strange and gooey oozing onto my face. It was like a horror movie, but I realised what it was and had a chuckle. I managed to seal the split with packing tape and I was able to cope with using it until a replacement arrived, even though the gel was rather depleted. Now I always make sure I have a spare mask, just in case!*

What about the hose?

The hose can be removed from the machine and cleaned when necessary. Disconnect it from the ventilator, and swish it in warm soapy water, in the same way as you would clean the mask. Wipe it over with a dry towel and hang it up to drain and dry out. Ensure that it is completely dry before re-connecting.

Clean the hose if you have had an infection, and regularly inspect it for any damage, splits or punctures.

Children and pets are very inquisitive and playful creatures so make sure they don't have access to your equipment. A pet's claws or teeth could easily puncture the hose or damage your mask, and a child's playful tug could dislodge the connections.

Should I wash my head gear & chin-strap in the washing machine?

Check your accessories' packaging for washing instructions. Unless otherwise stated, machine-washing and tumble-drying are not usually recommended, as they can weaken and damage velcro or plastic fastenings. This would increase the risk of air leaking from your mask, and you would also need to replace your items more frequently. Instead, wash them by hand in warm soapy water. Blot them in a towel to remove excess water, and hang them somewhere warm to dry.

In Brief

- Ensure all your equipment is set up in the correct position, making sure the power cord will not trip you up
- Read your manual. Ask for help if you need it
- Keep the ventilator free from dust; it needs very little cleaning
- Check filters often and replace as needed
- Keep mask and tubing clean, and check regularly for wear or damage
- Keep children and pets away from your equipment
- Take care when washing straps, chin-strap, head-cap
- If you suspect that your equipment has developed a fault contact your supplier or medical advisor immediately

CHAPTER 3

Using the Equipment

I had to be in Brompton Hospital for a week, to get used to the mask. It took a while, but one day my Consultant came in and said to me, "Just treat it as a friend," and I have never looked back.

VPAP user

Unless you've tried scuba diving, it probably seems strange to breathe into something covering your nose or face. Some people may experience initial feelings of claustrophobia, or even fear that the machine has now taken control of them. These feelings are usually soon overcome as the user gets accustomed to the sensation and becomes more confident.

Initially it may be helpful to spend short periods during the daytime wearing the mask with the machine switched on, while you are preoccupied listening to music, watching television, or reading. This can help you get 'acclimatised' to the equipment, and let you become familiar with fitting the mask comfortably on your face.

The first night I was rather scared of it and a nurse had to put the mask on me. During the second night I woke up, switched off the machine, took off the mask, and asked the nurse for a cup of tea. Suddenly I realised that the machine didn't control me – I controlled the machine! It was plain sailing after that.

After a period of adjustment sleeping with the machine becomes routine, and its benefits to your health will soon become apparent. As well as using your machine at night, don't forget it when you take a day-time nap. You need it whenever you sleep.

Minor problems sometimes occur at first such as a dry throat, sore skin or air leaks. Perhaps you can't get comfortable in bed, or worry that the noise of the equipment may disturb you. If the tips in this book cannot help you sort out your difficulty you should consult your Doctor or Respiratory Physician.

The two problems most widely reported by CPAP and ventilator users are air leaks around the mask, and damage to the facial skin. This chapter deals with air leaks, along with other common problems. See **Chapter 4 for Skincare**

How can I call to my family if I need them during the night?

In the early days of coping at home with the equipment, some people are worried in case they should need help from the family during the night, but fear the mask could prevent them from calling out loudly enough. If this is a concern of yours, you could put a baby monitor on your bedside table to enable you to summon help. Here's another simple solution which doesn't involve having to call out:

> *I equipped myself with a brass bell - the kind you see on a hotel reception desk. I've placed it within easy reach, and if I ever need help all I have to do is stretch out my hand and give it a big 'ding' to attract attention. I got mine at a very reasonable price, from an internet auction website. You know, I might never use it, but having it there, just in case, makes me feel much more confident.*

How do I choose the right mask for me?

It's important to feel comfortable with your mask and its head-cap or straps. There are several styles of mask. Some cover just the nose; others are full-face masks which go over both the nose and the mouth.

> *I felt swamped with a full mask covering nearly all my face, so I now use a small nasal mask.*

Also available are nasal-pillows which, unlike a mask, do not cover the entire nasal area. They consist of soft rubber or silicon plugs which seal the nose and hold tubes at the edge of the nostrils. There are various sizes, to allow for a good fit, and they are useful for people who develop soreness or damage to the facial tissue as they don't exert pressure on the face. Nasal-pillows may be preferable for those who get feelings of claustrophobia with the usual masks. They are also suitable for men with beards. Your choice will be guided by your Consultant's advice.

Masks are held in position by straps, harnesses or head-caps. Various factors have to be taken into account when choosing the correct type of mask and headgear to suit you, and it may initially take a little bit of trial and error to ensure a good fit.

As I am very small I have to use the smallest size of mask. I have a head-cap to keep the mask in position, and the hospital was able to supply me with a little head-cap which was specially made to fit my small head.

After you've had your mask for a while, don't be afraid to ask if you can try a different size or type if you are still having difficulties or discomfort.

I have tried three different types of mask, but always return to the full-face mask.

New products are coming onto the market all the time and you may wish to check for recent developments. For instance, there are now CPAP masks made from fabric. These are less likely to cause the pressure problems of the plastic versions, and they are available in a range of attractive colours. See **Appendix II Contacts List** for Equipment & Product Supplies.

I'm new to this and am having a problem positioning the straps

A mirror is useful at first, to help you position and fasten the straps correctly. Once you have adjusted them to a comfortable fit you'll probably need to undo only one strap in order to get the mask on and off, and you'll soon be able to do it without looking in the mirror.

If you've ever had your ears pierced you'll understand this. Remember how hard it was at first to put in your studs? It seemed impossible to find those tiny holes with a little sharp thing, even with a mirror, and you just kept on stabbing yourself! And then it all clicked into place and you could do it effortlessly, without even looking. In the same way, before you know it you'll be so proficient at putting on your mask that you'll wonder why you ever worried about it in the first place.

How can I stop air leaks?

Air leakage is a common problem, especially for a new NIV user. Noisy air leaks, or air blowing onto your eyes, can be rather irritating and may disturb your sleep. As you become used to adjusting your mask to fit correctly these disturbances should become fewer.

It's not essential to eliminate all leaks entirely. A small amount of leakage at the seal isn't a great problem, and won't decrease the benefits of the process. However, larger leaks can cause loud 'raspberry noises' and blow air onto the face or eyes. This is not only annoying but can affect the pressure of air getting to your air passages.

Here are a few suggestions that should help.

- ◆ The mask should be snug on your face, but not tight.
- ◆ Don't worry unduly about small leaks. You'll probably find they disappear of their own accord overnight, because your face tends to puff up slightly during sleep.
- ◆ Check that your straps or head-cap are not too large for you. You may need to try a smaller size, or to have a cap specially made for you if you have a small head.
- ◆ If an air leak occurs, gently tighten the straps but don't make them too tight. This can actually make things worse - if a strap is too tight it will make the opposite side of the mask lift up slightly, and this will cause yet another leak.
- ◆ If adjusting the straps doesn't work, lift the mask slightly off your face and then reposition it.
- ◆ Sometimes you'll get small leaks occurring during the night, when you move about in bed. If it bothers you, it may help to try a different sleeping position.
- ◆ Your pillow might dislodge the mask when you are sleeping on your side. See the next question in this chapter.

- Don't put face cream on the skin under your mask at bedtime as this can interfere with the seal and cause leaks. See **Chapter 4 Skincare**.

- Occasional small leaks can occur because the shape of your face changes when you lay down. The mask may be fine while you're in an upright position, but as soon as you lay down you get a small leak. Usually easily rectified with a minor adjustment to the straps.

I used to have problems when putting on my mask at bedtime. Little puffs of air would keep blowing into my eyes, and I'd sit up for ages, trying to sort it out by adjusting the straps. Then I discovered that if I just lay down and closed my eyes the leaks stopped. I guess it was because when my eyes were open the air was able to escape through the wrinkles!

- If the pressure on your machine is set too high it could slightly lift the mask off your skin, thus causing loud leaks. Your hospital unit will be able to check this and adjust pressure settings for you if needed.

- Check that your mask and tubing have no splits or punctures.

- If you've had your mask for a while it may need to be replaced.

- Check the fastenings on straps and head-gear - they do deteriorate over time, especially if washed in the washing machine, and they may be slipping during the night.

- Leaks can be caused by the weight of the hose pulling on the mask and dislodging it. Try to prevent the hose from slipping down by keeping it at your side on the bed, instead of letting it hang downwards. See also details of the Hose-Lift described further on in this chapter under "My arm gets caught up in the hose"

When I am lying on my side my mask gets pushed up by my pillow & I get air leaks

You may need to experiment in order to find a comfortable side position in which your pillow doesn't dislodge or distort the mask. If it gives enough support to your head, a softer pillow might suit. Try to mould a space along the edge of the pillow so that it doesn't dig into the mask. You could try using a smaller pillow, so that your mask and hose can hang over its edge.

> *My sleep was often disturbed because my CPAP mask got moved by my pillow when I lay on my side. Sometimes the mask got pressed onto my face which made me sore. But it was even worse when the mask got dislodged from my face as air escaped from it, and the machine couldn't deliver the continuous air pressure which I needed. By searching on the internet I managed to find an excellent pillow which is suitable for using with the mask, and it has eliminated my problems.*

Special pillows have been designed to be compatible with wearing a mask, and can be bought on-line or by mail order. They have strategically placed cut-outs on the left and right edges, into which your mask and hose will fit neatly. This prevents pressure on the mask and on your face, whatever position you sleep in. See **Appendix II Contacts List** for Equipment & Product Supplies.

My teeth hurt in the morning!

This is not as strange as it sounds. A mask strapped too tightly can put pressure on your mouth and teeth, making them feel uncomfortable. Check out the above tips for getting a comfortable fit.

> *Some mornings my face can be quite sore, and even my top teeth, if I've had my mask too tight.*

Even gentle pressure from your mask can cause pain when you have tooth decay or gum disease. Dental hygiene is therefore important in order to avoid this problem: brush your teeth every day, and don't miss your regular dental check-ups.

I have a moustache: will it get in the way of my mask?

A beard or moustache sometimes complicates matters by preventing the mask from fitting closely to the face. This can be a cause of leaks, so do keep facial hair neatly trimmed. Nasal-pillows, rather than a full-face or nasal mask, may be a better choice for people with facial hair.

My arm gets caught up in the hose while I'm asleep: also the hose sometimes falls down, pulling the mask & causing air leaks

There is a gadget called a Hose-Lift which has been designed to remedy this particular problem. It consists of a flat base section, and a tall lightweight mast assembly with a loop at the top. The base slips under the mattress to hold the mast in place at the head of the bed, and your hose is threaded through the loop. This supports the hose and holds it above your head, so you can't get caught up in it. If you move in your sleep it will swing over with you, preventing you from getting entangled. It is light-weight and easily assembled, so you can take it with you when you travel without any fuss.

Another benefit of the Hose-Lift is that it supports the weight of the hose and prevents it from falling down off the bed. This relieves the drag of the hose on the mask, which in turn decreases pressure marks and soreness on the face, and reduces air leaks at the top of the mask. See **Appendix II Contacts List** for Equipment & Product Supplies.

Some people have considered screwing a hook or plant-pot holder on the wall above their bed, so that they can hang up their hose there. THIS REALLY IS NOT A GOOD IDEA. Although your hose will be supported, it will not move from side to side when you change your sleeping position, so it could get tugged and pulled from its connections. Tension on the hose could lift the mask off your face, causing leaks. It may even pull down the hanging fixture, if it's not adequately fastened to the wall.

In addition, there is a REAL DANGER OF THE HOSE GETTING WRAPPED TIGHTLY AROUND YOUR NECK. Do not risk it. Medical products such as the Hose-Lift have been specially designed to do the job safely. They are reasonably priced and readily available.

Should you experience drops of condensation (or rain-out) forming in the hose while it is suspended above you please refer to the section on Humidifiers in **Chapter 2 Care of Your Equipment**.

My mouth doesn't stay closed while I sleep

If your mouth stays open air can escape, and your machine may not function as efficiently because the pressure of the air it delivers to you will be reduced. Also secretions can leak from your mouth making your lips sore and leaving a residue around them.

One remedy is to use a full-face mask rather than a nasal mask. This will cover both your mouth and the nasal area, so having an open mouth will not be such a problem. You may need to try different styles or sizes of mask in order to get a comfortable fit.

If you prefer a nasal mask, then using a chin-strap should help keep your mouth closed. The basic style of chin-strap consists of a band of soft, washable fabric. Position it under your chin, bring the two ends up around your head, and secure them neatly on top with the velcro fastener. The strap will gently hold your jaw closed, but you can still open your mouth if you need to. Your hospital unit is usually able to supply you with one of these, or you may know a seamstress who could make one for you.

Restless sleepers sometimes report difficulties with this type of chin-strap as it could slip off when they toss and turn during the night. In this situation other, more elaborate, styles of chin-strap may be more suitable. There are chin-straps with an additional support strap around the back or front of the head to hold them firmly in position. Some also have a rounded cup-shape section to hold the chin. You can buy them on-line and by mail order. See **Appendix II Contacts List** for Equipment & Product Supplies.

I had problems because my mouth stayed open. My hospital unit gave me a chin-strap but it just wouldn't stay in place, so I bought a better one on the internet. It stays firmly in position even if I toss and turn, and I'm very pleased with it.

Studies suggest that, over time, patients often do learn to position their tongue and soft palate in such a way that their air pathway to the lungs, via the nose, is maintained, thus cutting down on air leaking through the mouth. However, patients who have had surgery on the soft palate, (such as a UPPP operation to reduce snoring,) may find it harder to do this, and for them a chin-strap or a full-face mask may be the answer.

If secretions from the mouth continue to be a problem try tucking a small linen handkerchief, or a piece of muslin, into the front of the chin-strap to mop up any moisture. Rinse it out with a little soap and water in the morning.

My throat gets sore at night

Some people experience a dry or sore throat when they first have to use Non-Invasive Ventilation. Often they will find that these symptoms go away once they have become accustomed to using the equipment, but occasionally the sensations persist.

To remedy this problem your Consultant may recommend that you use a humidifier along with your machine. The humidifier warms and moistens the air that you breathe in, and relieves the uncomfortable feelings. The apparatus contains a small reservoir of distilled water, so be very careful to set it up in a position where it cannot get knocked, to avoid any danger of water getting into your other equipment.

I have placed my Nippy higher than the Humidifier now. They used to be side-by-side, but one day I knocked the table, water got into my Nippy and it blew the fuse.

See **Chapter 2 Care of Your Equipment** Also consult the hand-book supplied with your humidifier.

During the normal process of breathing, air is usually inhaled through the nose, where it is warmed and moistened before entering the lungs. A person who breathes through the mouth misses out on this warming process. In addition, if they are receiving air under pressure through the NIV machine, the dryness or discomfort in the mouth, nose or throat can be further aggravated. A patient who uses a full-face mask and breathes through the mouth may experience these feelings too, and they also could find it helpful to use a humidifier.

To ease a dry nose or nasal passages, if you are not using a humidifier, you may find a light application of cream helpful. Use the cream specially formulated for use with NIV masks. See **Appendix II Contacts List**. Do not use a petroleum based product as this can damage your mask.

My nose gets cold

All the while you are using your equipment, air is being passed under pressure to your nose, and this can make your nose or face feel cold. Raising the temperature in your bedroom would help.

Insulation around the hose can help too. As air travels through the length of the hose its temperature can drop. The insulation will help to reduce this and your nose may not get so cold. You can insulate the hose by wrapping it with something like bubble-wrap or fleecy fabric, or by using a purpose-made cover called a Tube Wrap. For suppliers see **Appendix II Contacts List**

> *My Tube Wrap only cost a few pounds and was easy to fit. I just had to slip it onto the hose and fasten it with a little popper. I've definitely noticed the difference, because I rarely have a cold nose in the morning now.*

The straps leave marks on my cheeks

Tight straps can leave impression marks on your face, but they do eventually fade during the day. Although harmless, they can make some people feel self-conscious, especially if some well-meaning person draws attention to it, saying, "You must have been lying on something!" In the morning gently massage the marks with a moisturising skin cream to help ease the indentations.

To prevent or reduce these impression marks you should ensure that you do not over-tighten the straps, and also make sure that the hose is not pulling on the mask. Some of the tips already mentioned above may be of help. If the problem persists try placing padding of some sort, such as cotton wool (absorbent cotton) pads, under the straps. Use thin padding. If it's too thick the mask won't be able to make an efficient air-tight seal with your face, and you'll get air leaks.

> *I cut up the shoulder pads from old garments, and use them under the straps. They work very well.*

Soft, fleecy Cheek Strap covers are sold by specialist equipment suppliers. They are available in several sizes and colours. See **Appendix II Contacts List**.

What should I do if there's a power cut in the night?

This is something which you must discuss with your Consultant or medical advisor, in case this situation arises. They can tell you whether or not it is safe for you to sleep without your machine. Each person's condition is different, so you must be guided by your own medical team.

The machine's alarm will sound off to alert and wake you, if you are using it when the power goes off. However, if your equipment stops working, but your power supply is fine, then there's probably a fault with your machine. Contact your machine's supplier immediately so that a replacement can be arranged.

If you experience a night-time power failure in your area, telephone your electricity supplier and ask how long they expect the power to be off. If the delay will be prolonged, and you have been advised not to sleep without the equipment, you may need to make other sleeping arrangements, such as taking your machine to a friend's home so that you can sleep there for the rest of the night. It's a good idea to have your arrangements already in place, in case of such a situation.

During a prolonged power failure my GP arranged for me to go into my local hospital overnight, rather than send me to my specialist Respiratory Support Unit which is eighty miles away. The ambulance people didn't know what to expect when they arrived at my house. They'd been told that the patient was on a ventilator, and I think they expected me to be in an iron lung or something! At the hospital I was put onto a general ward for the night, but I didn't get to bed very quickly as I had to spend ages explaining my ventilator to curious staff members who had never seen one before.

Contact your specialist unit if you are in any doubt. Arrangements will be made for you to be admitted to the nearest hospital overnight if it is considered necessary. If **at any time** you are admitted to hospital ensure that your ventilator is taken with you. The ward staff there may not be familiar with your equipment, or know how it works. If that is the case, they should contact your specialist unit for information.

Some electricity supply companies have a Priority User scheme for customers who rely on essential medical equipment such as ventilators or dialysis machines. Customers can register under this scheme and will be given, as far as possible, priority for restoring their supply in the event of a power failure. Advance notice will be given to the registered customers when the company plans any work in the area which could lead to temporary cuts in their customers' domestic power supply. Check with your own electricity supplier.

In Brief

- ◆ It's normal to feel strange when first using the mask. These feelings are usually overcome very quickly
- ◆ The correct size and style of mask will help prevent air leaks and skin ulceration
- ◆ A beard or moustache may cause air leaks by preventing the mask from making a good fit. The use of nasal-pillows instead of nasal or full-face masks may solve this problem
- ◆ The mask should not be too tight on the face
- ◆ Additional equipment such as a chin-strap, the Hose-Lift and special pillows can increase comfort at night
- ◆ Find out whether you may safely sleep without the machine for a few hours in an emergency. Make contingency plans to sleep elsewhere in case of a power cut.
- ◆ Don't forget you need the equipment whenever you sleep, day or night. If you didn't get to sleep at night because of a power failure, and are catching up on some shut-eye next day, make sure you use your machine.
- ◆ Talk to your medical advisor if you experience difficulties in using your equipment or if it causes you any discomfort

CHAPTER 4

Skin Care

The skin is the largest organ of the body. It protects you, heals itself and lasts a lifetime. Your skin works hard to keep you healthy, and you can return the favour by taking care of it.

NHS UK

This chapter is about taking care of your face, and how to avoid mask-related abrasions or damage to the facial skin and its underlying tissue. These kinds of problems are often reported by NIV users, but they can be reduced or prevented with care.

Irritated or reddened skin on the face is a common concern. Damaged areas of skin could become sore, and you may feel rather self-conscious because of red patches on your face. A new NIV user may find that the mask makes their face a little sore at first, until they get accustomed to it and have learned how to fit it comfortably. If a problem persists or reappears don't neglect it. By dealing with it as soon as possible you can avoid further problems arising - prevention is better than cure. This chapter offers advice for preventing skin damage as well as dealing with it, should it become necessary.

Although our skin carries bacteria, yeasts and other micro-organisms, it is a highly effective self-repairing barrier against infections, unless it is damaged or exposed to sunlight. Skin care for your face is therefore very important so that soreness and broken skin do not lead to difficulties in using your equipment.

I'm a man - surely I needn't bother with skincare?

Skincare is important for both men and women. In fact men may have to take additional care, because of beard growth and shaving. So, men, it is important for you to take care of your skin too! Broken skin is not macho and can be painful! You can try any of the products mentioned in this chapter, or purchase products specially formulated for men. For example, a leading skin-care company makes a wide range of shaving and skin products for men, including creams which help to reduce blemishes and redness. They are allergy tested and fragrance free. You can often obtain advice and even a free trial sample at in-store cosmetics counters.

How can I prevent the mask making my face sore?

To prevent soreness you should first make sure that your mask is a good fit, and is snug but not tight on your face. Don't over-tighten the straps. If they are too tight they will leave marks on your face and put pressure on the mask. This can increase moisture and friction which will damage your skin, for instance on the bridge of the nose. Bear in mind that facial tissue tends to puff up slightly during sleep, so your mask becomes tighter by the morning.

> *The mask has caused reddening and soreness of the nose and cheeks and in my case produces acne-type spots. My Doctor has prescribed Metrogel.*

Sometimes a mask can contribute to irritation or breakdown of the skin but these problems don't always need medications. Metrogel is prescribed to treat Rosacea. This is a condition in which the cheeks and nose have a flushed appearance because of enlarged facial blood vessels. Perhaps it may be aggravated by the mask, but is not caused by it.

Oils and bacteria from your face will build up on your mask. These can affect your skin, and could also perish the plastic parts of the mask, unless you are careful about keeping it clean. Skin creams can have a similar damaging effect, although specialist creams are available which can be used with the equipment and are not harmful to the mask. See **Appendix II Contacts List**. Be careful though: creams and lotions make the skin slippery, and can cause air leaks by preventing the mask from making a good air-tight seal.

Gently cleanse your face of any cosmetics or grime each evening before using your mask. Remember that when you're using the machine there should not be any cream on the parts of your face where the mask touches. Therefore, if you want to moisturise your skin in the evening it would be advisable to do so at least an hour or more before going to bed, so that the product is absorbed into your skin before you put on the mask.

Or use one of the specialist creams mentioned above.

To keep your mask free of contamination it should be cleaned regularly. This is particularly important if you have infections or skin problems such as coughs, colds, cold sores, Rosacea or Acne.

For tips on getting a good fit and keeping the mask clean see **Chapter 2 Care of Your Equipment** & **Chapter 3 Using the Equipment**.

Can I use ordinary soap on my face?

Cleanse your face gently using either a simple cleansing lotion or mild soap. Pat the skin dry, don't rub, and apply a gentle moisturiser.

Aqueous Cream BP is a cheap and excellent product which is obtainable without prescription from your Pharmacist. This non-greasy cream can be used as a moisturising skin cream and, if mixed with water, it also makes an excellent soap-free skin cleanser which is suitable for face or body.

> *I use Aqueous Cream as a cleanser and as a moisturiser for my face and the dry skin on other parts of my body. I buy a big tub and transfer a small amount into a little plastic pot for ease of use. It's much easier to handle than the big tub, and better for taking into the shower. It's also an ideal size for popping into my wash bag when travelling.*

What about moisturising?

There is no need to spend a lot of money on products – the Aqueous Cream mentioned above works well for day-time moisturising. Large supermarkets sell their own ranges of fragrance-free creams and soaps, and other simple products are available there. A light application of lip salve or skin cream will help if your lips tend to get dry overnight, but make sure it is not petroleum-based.

It is not advisable to use Petroleum Jelly on your face as it is not absorbed into the skin and prevents the natural evaporation of moisture from your face. If it gets transferred to your mask it could perish the plastic.

For suppliers of non-petroleum-based skin creams, suitable for use with a mask, see **Appendix II Contacts List**. These creams may be used to relieve soreness inside the nostrils, as well as on the face.

Please note: Petroleum-based creams and lotions should NOT be used when using Oxygen Therapy as there is a risk of burn damage to the skin.

Should I stay out of the sun?

Sunshine can be good for your health, but with precautions. Sunlight contains potentially damaging Ultra Violet (UV) rays, and although it helps our bodies make vitamin D, an essential vitamin, over-exposure can damage our skin, eyes and hair. So it's important for everyone to protect their skin when out in the sun.

Your facial skin in particular may be more delicate because you are using a mask, so you'll need to protect it well. Always apply a sun-block cream when you are out in the sun and remember to reapply regularly, especially after swimming. A sun hat and sun glasses are also advised, and a beach umbrella is always a good idea especially when you're on holiday in a hot climate. A champion bodybuilder says:

> *If you have delicate, thin skin (like bodybuilders do during competitions), or if your skin is tattooed, you can easily get sun damage. I recommend the use of High Factor Baby Sun Block products.*

This is a great tip! Sunscreen products for babies and children are excellent for delicate skin, and have a very high Sun Protection Factor (SPF).

If you spend time outdoors, whether or not the sun is shining, it's a good idea to routinely use skin creams which have SPF ingredients incorporated into them, to protect against UV rays. Many popular face creams do contain this; check the label when purchasing. It is not advisable to use sun beds or tanning booths. Get further information and advice about sun damage from The Cancer Research organisation. See **Appendix II Contacts List**

I am embarrassed by the red patches on my face

> *One thing that I really feel embarrassed about is my nose which is sometimes really red, but I don't know of any products to help with this.*

Fortunately most people's problems are minor and can be quickly dealt with. However, some find that pressure from the mask gives rise to frequent red patches on their face. They worry about other people noticing it, and this can make them feel self-conscious, and can lower their self-esteem.

Cosmetic creams which camouflage redness are available. They have a green base, but don't worry - they are not actually green and will not make you look like a cartoon character. The green ingredient just neutralises and tones down the redness of your skin.

Apply it sparingly with a make-up sponge or finger-tip, gently dabbing it where required. If you find it too thick, try mixing it with a tiny spot of your usual moisturiser or day-cream, to make it easier to apply. If you wear make-up put the concealer cream on first, before applying your cosmetics.

The initial cost for this kind of product may seem a bit expensive, but if you use only a small amount each time the tube will last for ages. There are several shades to choose from, so you can buy one to match your own skin tone. Some cream foundation products are available in shades suitable for darker skin tones. They may not contain the green ingredient but do help conceal blemishes.

I was asked to address a local women's group, but being aware of the redness of my face, and feeling very self-conscious, I was tempted to refuse. A friend recommended I try a green-based foundation cream. It was excellent and did the trick - my face didn't look red anymore. I made my presentation to the group, it went very well, and I was confident enough to take on further speaking engagements.

My face is very sore

If your facial skin becomes very sore or broken you may need to cover the affected area at night to prevent discomfort from the mask. It's not a good idea to use a sticking plaster/band-aid because when you remove it in the morning you could easily damage other parts of the delicate skin, making things worse. A piece of low adherent dressing, held in position by microporous surgical tape, would be a better option. Both are obtainable at Pharmacies and some supermarkets.

Some people use a cotton wool (absorbent cotton) pad to cushion the bridge of the nose. Split the pad in half and use one piece, making sure the smooth side is placed against your skin.

In more severe cases, if the facial tissue is damaged, a Doctor or Practice Nurse should be able to provide a suitable dressing on prescription, such as Granuflex. Whatever you use, try to ensure that it is not so thick that it causes air leakage.

I have been given a supply of an adhesive cotton flannelette dressing. It sticks onto the mask so that the soft cotton side cushions my face. It works very well and doesn't damage the mask.

Mask Comfort Liners are now available from commercial companies. Made from naturally absorbent fibres, they protect the skin and allow for the use of night-time facial skincare products. Their use will also help keep the mask free from contamination. Each liner is intended for a single use only, but with care could be used twice.

You may feel that the cost of these liners is too expensive for regular daily use, but perhaps would consider them cost-effective as a useful temporary measure to relieve severe skin soreness. See **Appendix II Contacts List** for Medical Equipment Suppliers

In rare cases an allergic reaction to the plastic/latex in the mask can develop. If you think this has happened to you should consult your Doctor or the specialist hospital unit. Don't delay in contacting them for advice if your face becomes so sore that you find it painful to use your mask.

Excellent relief from pressure marks, redness and soreness has been reported with the use of a 'Hose-Lift'. This device holds the hose and supports its weight, which stops it from pulling on the mask. See **Chapter 3 Using the Equipment** – "My arm gets caught up in the hose".

Would Vitamin Supplements help my skin?

Bear in mind that good skin care also comes from within. Essential vitamins, minerals and plenty of fluids are required in order to maintain the skin's healthy condition. Vitamin A, for example, helps maintain healthy skin and strengthens the immune system. It's found in foods such as full-fat dairy products, oily fish, spinach, peppers, watercress, and dried apricots. Vegetable oils, wheatgerm, seeds and nuts provide Vitamin E which helps prevent cell damage and also boosts the immune system. Riboflavin is also important; it's in milk, eggs, rice, mushrooms and fortified breakfast cereals.

The best way to get your daily vitamins and minerals is from a balanced diet. Your "Five-a-Day Fruit & Veg" is a good starting point. For healthy eating tips see **Chapter 13 Diet & Nutrition**. If you take vitamin supplements be aware that there are dangers associated with exceeding the Recommended Daily Allowance (RDA) so always read the packet, and don't be tempted to take more than the recommended dose.

In Brief

- Avoid future problems by taking care of your skin
- Ensure your mask fits well. Keep it clean
- Gently cleanse & moisturise your face
- Avoid sun damage: use sun block cream
- Specialist cosmetics can disguise redness
- Eat a good, varied diet and don't forget your fluids
- Seek the help of your Doctor if skin problems do not respond to the simple treatments described here

CHAPTER 5

General Health Issues

Night after night brings me grief. When I lie down to sleep, the hours drag. I toss all night and long for dawn.

Job 7:3-4 Good News Bible

Nights can be very stressful for those with untreated sleep-disordered breathing problems, and lack of refreshing sleep (as well as the respiratory condition) can affect your general health.

After a bad night it's difficult to get through the day when you're feeling so tired or exhausted. Failure to breathe efficiently causes yet more tiredness, and brings additional problems. With low oxygen levels and a high concentration of carbon dioxide in the blood, there can be symptoms such as headaches, visual disturbances, and poor muscle tone. You may feel cold, and need extra clothing or heating to keep you cosy.

Once you start on NIV therapy these symptoms will be reduced, or even eliminated entirely, as your ventilation equipment normalises your blood gases levels.

Before I had the ventilator I used to get dreadful headaches and sickness in the mornings, but these symptoms are gone. I also used to have frequent chest infections, but they are rare now, so any hassle from using the machine is well worth it, in order to stay well.

NIV keeps blood gases at more normal levels, and the patient's daytime function improves. A ventilator helps reduce the work and fatigue of the respiratory muscles and allows sleep to be more refreshing. For CPAP users, their machine helps them to have nights uninterrupted by snoring and sleep disturbances. Sleep partners start to feel the benefits too because the quality of their own sleep will be improved once their partner's snoring and restlessness is reduced.

As mentioned in **Chapter 7 Your Emotions & You** it's good to be in tune with your body, so that you are aware of your own state of health and know when to be concerned. It's one of the ways you can be pro-active in caring for yourself and your medical needs.

This chapter covers some general topics such as nasal congestion at night, bloating, and sensitivity to household chemicals. Other health-related topics are covered elsewhere in this book. For example:

- Dental pain (Chapter 3)
- Sore or red face (Chapter 4)
- Travelling by air (Chapter 6)
- Diet & Nutrition (Chapter 13)
- Smoking (Chapter 14)
- Exercise (Chapter 15)
- Shortness of breath whilst swimming (Chapter 15)
- Dealing with negative emotions (Chapter 10)

Here are some things you can do to help yourself stay as healthy as possible:

- Avoid places that are smoky and don't smoke yourself
- Learn to recognise anything that affects you adversely, and take steps to avoid or deal with it in future
- Form a good relationship with your doctor and take prescribed medications as directed
- Coughs, colds, asthma and other common problems should be treated effectively
- Avoid people with heavy colds
- Very important and worth repeating – Don't Smoke
- Try to remain active, within your own capabilities, and do gentle exercise if you can
- Eat nutritious foods. Seek advice if your weight is a problem

- People with respiratory or lung conditions are considered to be in a high risk category when it comes to influenza, and therefore should seriously consider having annual Flu Vaccinations
- Pneumonia vaccinations are also available; ask for advice from your Physician
- Deal promptly with any problems arising from using your mask or equipment

How can I deal with a blocked nose?

The common cold is the usual cause of a blocked or runny nose. Similar symptoms can be caused by a reaction to pollen, perfumes or household chemicals. See "I Am Sensitive to Household Perfumes and Chemicals" in this chapter, and **Chapter 11 Sensitivity to Indoor Pollution.** See **Appendix II Contacts List** for organisations which offer useful advice on allergies and hay fever.

Some people find that dairy foods can affect their nasal passages

I don't eat dairy products in the evening as they seem to increase the formation of mucus and make me feel 'bunged up' during the night.

Ordinarily, for most people a cold or blocked nose is nothing more than an inconvenience, but users of NIV may find it rather tricky to use their machine.

If you can clear your nose before switching on, you'll probably find that the air flow provided by the equipment will keep the nasal passages clear, and you'll be able to get some sleep. A quick sniff with a menthol nasal inhaler, or other congestion relief medication, may be all you need before going to bed, but be careful of overuse. Nasal decongestants, if used too frequently, may result in headache and increased congestion. Antihistamine tablets can be useful too, depending on the actual cause of your nasal congestion. Whichever product you use, it is advisable to ask the advice of your Doctor or Pharmacist, in case there are contra-indications for your condition.

Hydration is important when you have congestion - have plenty to drink as fluids help to keep mucus thinner and less sticky

Massage can help to clear sinus passages. It's simple to do, and you can do it to yourself. Place two fingers on the sinus area and move your fingertips round in a circular motion using gentle pressure. Do this around the nose, and on the forehead above the nose.

Simple steam inhalation sessions can help with nasal congestion. Fill a bowl with hot water till about one-third full. Lean over the bowl and pull a towel over your head and the bowl. Inhale the steam for a few minutes. This will help to loosen the mucus in the lungs, nose and throat, and make it easier to clear. You must take precautions to avoid scalding yourself with the hot water. Children should not carry out steam inhalation unless they are supervised by an adult.

Inhaling the steam in the bathroom, when you're running the hot bath water or taking a shower, can also help.

Another home remedy for relieving congestion is to snort warm, slightly salty water into your nose. Some people use boiled, cooled water and a tiny pinch of salt, and you can also buy products for this purpose. Ask your Doctor for advice. Do NOT use salt water if your nose is sensitive, as you may aggravate the nasal tissues. Seek medical advice if the symptoms persist.

For a chesty congestion, hot drinks may help to loosen the mucus. Congestion can also sometimes be helped by 'tipping-up'. Tipping-up is postural drainage of the airways using gravity.

> *I sometimes get congestion in my lungs so to clear it I 'tip-up'. For this my head needs to be lower than my body so I lie over the end of my bed or over an arm of the sofa, with my head hanging down towards the floor, or I lie on pillows on the bed. You have to do one side at a time, so I always start with the side that feels worse in case the process makes me too tired to do both sides. This is what I do – I lie on my least affected side. Then I proceed to tap with the palm of my hand on the other side. (My partner sometimes helps here). It has to be done firmly, but not hard, in a percussive manner, to loosen the secretions and enable them to shift. Once the secretions reach my upper airways I can try to cough them up. Then I do the other side, if I feel up to it.*

If these simple measures do not help, and the congestion worsens or does not improve within three days, you should consult your Physician. Do not delay in seeking help if you are having difficulties in using your ventilation equipment.

Never be tempted to lie down, or go to sleep, with a cough lozenge or throat pastille in your mouth. This is very dangerous as the lozenge could be moved by the air-flow of your equipment, and get lodged in your windpipe.

Surprisingly, perhaps, some people report getting fewer colds once they start using NIV therapy. With the assisted ventilation treatment they no longer suffer from sleep deprivation and low blood oxygen levels. As a result their immune system starts to function better, and they experience fewer coughs, colds and cold sores.

I've been suffering from bloating

Bloating occurs when air is forced into the digestive system, via the oesophagus, instead of entering the airway (Aerophagia). Air fills the stomach and digestive tract, and causes distension. This produces flatulence, which can be embarrassing as well as uncomfortable.

When I first had my Nippy machine I suffered from wind and bloating, but this seems to have settled down.

This may be a problem for patients new to using a ventilator. Once they have become accustomed to using the machine the bloating usually diminishes. It's worth trying out different sleeping positions to see which is less likely to make you swallow the air.

If bloating does persist, then the pressure settings on your equipment may need to be reduced. Talk to your hospital unit and they will do the adjustments, or they may ask you to try out a different type of ventilator.

What about alcohol? I like to have a drink with my mates

Many people enjoy a glass of wine with dinner, or the occasional pint of beer, and they do not experience any problems. However alcohol, or a drug such as a sedative or pain-relief medication, makes the muscles of the upper airway relax more than normal. This increases the risk of the airways collapsing and becoming blocked during sleep. If you have Sleep Apnoea, or other sleep disordered respiratory condition, be aware of this side-effect. Take care to limit your alcohol intake, and avoid the routine use of medications unless prescribed by your Doctor. Never combine alcohol with sedating drugs.

Over-indulgence of alcohol and drugs also makes it harder for the brain to register that there is a lack of oxygen in the body. This could cause longer and more serious pauses in breathing, perhaps to the point of being unable to rouse yourself from sleep if you stop breathing. During certain stages of sleep muscle tone is very relaxed, almost like being paralysed, which is not good for people who already have difficulty in breathing unaided whilst asleep. Falling asleep, or passing out, without first connecting to your ventilator, can obviously have very serious implications.

If you do remember to connect to your ventilator, but are in a drunken state, there is a danger that you may vomit into the mask. The air pressure can force the vomit back down into the airway passage, and this can be extremely dangerous, especially if you are too inebriated to rouse yourself.

My GP doesn't know much about my condition or equipment and can't give me advice

Bear in mind that your Doctor's knowledge may be limited in this specialized subject. Any advice offered to you will be based on this limited knowledge, and on the experiences of his other patients, but those patients may well have had experiences which are not the same as your own. Therefore the advice of one Doctor may differ from the advice of another and it's up to you to help your own medical practitioner understand about your particular condition.

If you are served by a large medical practice, and see a different Doctor each time you visit, there may not be the same continuity of care as in the days of the 'Family Doctor'. Your particular history may not be familiar to the Doctor who sees you, and they'll have to check through, and try to understand, your copious medical records. Therefore, as mentioned earlier in this chapter, it's important to be aware of your own state of health, so you can help the Doctor with relevant information. If necessary, phone your hospital care team for advice.

There are eight Doctors at my Health Centre. The patients do not get a choice of which one to see, so I cannot see the same one every time, and consequently none of them is very familiar with me or my problems. When I went there with a chest infection the Doctor who saw me remarked that my breathing was very bad. I told him that I have to use a ventilator for my respiratory failure, and that it was all in my notes. He told me he didn't have time to read my notes, and said I'd better phone the hospital!

My Doctor doesn't understand the difference between CPAP & my Ventilator

There are several types of NIV machine, and although they are used for a range of differing respiratory disorders, they all involve similar masks and accessories. So, it's not surprising that the subject can be confusing to anyone who doesn't have specialist knowledge or experience. Perhaps you can help by giving your Doctors the information they need.

I was admitted to hospital to sleep overnight when there was a power-cut at home. In the morning I overheard a Ward Sister in the corridor telling the nurses that my machine was a CPAP to treat Sleep Apnoea. I popped my head out of the door and told her she was incorrect – it was actually a Nippy ventilator for mechanical respiratory assistance. They all came into my room, and I was able to demonstrate the Nippy to them and answer all their questions. It was the first time they had seen one.

A common mistake made by doctors, nurses and dentists. is the assumption that all patients who use NIV have Sleep Apnoea. The use of CPAP machines to alleviate Sleep Apnoea and snoring problems is now widely known to the general public and medical practitioners. Less well-known, however, is the use of Non-Invasive Ventilation for other respiratory disorders. As mentioned above, confusion can arise because similar designs of mask may be used for both types of equipment. Sometimes the equipment is mistaken for a nebuliser, with the assumption that the patient has Asthma.

> *Because my medical notes showed that I use a ventilator, my Doctor assumed that it was a CPAP for Sleep Apnoea. He didn't quite understand the difference, so in the end I took my Nippy along to his office, demonstrated its function and explained how it differed from a CPAP.*

Some medical personnel don't seem to understand my condition

> *I haven't had to explain my condition to my GP but when it comes to the general ward in hospital I can say YES – it is like a stuck record!*

You must take your ventilator with you if admitted to hospital. Unless you are in your specialist Lung Function ward, the Doctors and nursing staff who are looking after you may not be fully aware of your condition or be familiar with your equipment. See also **Chapter 3 Using the Equipment**. If you are there for a problem which is not related to your respiratory condition, don't be afraid to let the medical team know the details. Ask questions if you feel that your treatment may not be appropriate, and suggest they contact your Consultant for further details.

> *I've had to explain my condition to various Doctors, and on four occasions I have given a talk to small groups of medical students.*

Being well informed about your own health means you will be able to help the members of your medical treatment team who are unfamiliar with your particular condition.

- Perhaps you are unable to hold your breath for more than a few seconds, or your breathing is restricted if you lie in a certain position. When having an X-ray or scan it is important to explain this to the Radiologist, so that together you can find a suitable compromise.

- If you are booking a hypnotherapy session, tell the therapist about your breathing or sleeping disorder.

- Let your Dental Surgeon know about it when you arrive for your appointment so that you can be allowed time to get seated comfortably, in a position that doesn't restrict your breathing. See the next question should you require a general anaesthetic for dental surgery.

Would I have difficulties during surgery?

Surgical procedures using general anaesthesia have to be carefully planned in order to deal with any existing ventilatory problems. If you are considering a surgical operation, it is **very important** to mention your condition to your Surgeon and the medical team at the onset of discussions. You must let them know the extent of your difficulties, and give them contact details of your Respiratory Consultant so that they can confer. Your Surgeon and Consultant will work together to ensure all goes well, and your Anaesthetist will be fully briefed.

I needed a gall-bladder operation and the Surgeon was very cautious because of my breathing problems. However he got in touch with my respiratory specialist who gave advice on how to deal with me, and the operation went ahead. They have all sorts of high-tech equipment these days and my ventilation was taken care of. Everything went very well and there were no complications.

Some operations can be performed under a local or epidural anaesthetic.

When my hysterectomy was performed I had an epidural as I have Sleep Apnoea, and a general anaesthetic was considered to be a risk.

I am sensitive to household chemicals & perfumes

Many people these days report increased sensitivity to common household products, perfumes, dust and moulds, whether or not they have an underlying medical condition.

Perfumes and certain chemicals do affect me by making me cough. If I want to use a fragrance I use natural oils.

It may be difficult to avoid these things, especially in other people's houses, but there are precautions you can take to minimise exposure in your own home. Advice can be found on the British Lung Foundation website. See **Appendix II Contacts List**. Also see **Chapter 11 Sensitivity to Indoor Pollution** which has useful tips.

What else could have an effect on my breathing?

It's not possible to generalise as we are all different, but the following points have been mentioned:

- ◆ Avoid a heavy evening meal close to bedtime. For some people a full stomach can restrict their lung capacity

I can eat only small meals because I soon get uncomfortably full, and it affects my breathing.

- ◆ Certain medications can affect breathing. It's very important to read the information leaflets, and report any side effects to your Doctor

One night I woke in the early hours, having difficulty breathing on my ventilator. I phoned the Respiratory Support Unit at my hospital for advice. When I mentioned that I had just started to take an anti-inflammatory medication prescribed by my GP, they told me to stop taking the tablets and go back to my Doctor in the morning for a different drug.

Chapter 5: General Health Issues

- Some people find it harder to breathe in very hot, cold, or windy weather

The wind seems to take my breath away! Change of temperature, just going from a warm room to a cold one, can affect my breathing.

- Shortness of breath can occur in times of stress or anxiety. It's important to try to stay calm. See **Chapter 10 Dealing With The Feelings**

- When you lie on your back, gravity pulls on the soft tissues at the back of the throat and in your neck. This can cause the upper airway passage to become narrow, which affects your breathing and aggravates Sleep Apnoea. These symptoms may be improved if you sleep on one side, rather than on your back. Try putting pillows against your back to prop yourself on your side

- Being overweight can increase the risk of sleep-disordered breathing. See **Chapter 13 Diet & Nutrition**

This might seem a strange question, but my toenails have changed. Could my condition be to blame?

Respiratory conditions and poor circulation can sometimes have an effect on finger and toe nails, because of lower oxygen levels in the blood. This may slow the growth of nails and cause them to thicken. Yellow discolouration can be the result of this slow growth and thickening. Quite often the nail on the big toe (or Hallux) is the most affected.

It's a harmless side effect although rather unattractive. However, if the nails are causing discomfort when you're wearing shoes, there is a remedy. Thickened nails can be treated painlessly by a Chiropodist or Podiatrist who will reduce the thickness using an electric chiropody drill with a sanding disc.

Injury or fungal infections can also cause changes to the nails. If you are at all concerned, consult your Doctor or Chiropodist. Foot care is particularly important if you are diabetic.

In Brief

- Pay attention to your own body and health; deal with health problems effectively, as soon as you notice them; seek advice if necessary
- Follow a healthy life-style
- Don't smoke
- Some prescription drugs can affect breathing. Always read the information leaflet supplied with your medicines.
- Keep the use of alcohol and non-prescription drugs to a minimum
- Deal with indoor pollutants such as smoke, chemicals and perfumes
- Be prepared to inform Doctors and other health care workers about your condition and equipment. This is very important if you have to undergo a surgical operation
- Seek early medical advice if you experience breathing difficulties

CHAPTER 6

Travel

Advance preparation can save you a lot of time and effort in the long run. It is far easier to deal with any problems from home, than in a foreign country where you may have to deal with language barriers.

Flying With Disability

Travelling with your ventilation equipment, especially when going abroad, has practical considerations which have to be addressed. For foreign travel, security rules at airports and ports can be strict, and you should make advance arrangements for your equipment to be allowed through Passport Control. Don't forget arrangements for the return trip too.

Always make contact well in advance of your trip, and check things out at your point of departure and arrival, as well as any transfers. Take letters from your doctor/hospital with details of your condition and equipment, translated into the language of your holiday destination, to produce if requested. If you plan to take any prescribed or over-the-counter medications with you see below "Do I need to carry a letter from my Doctor?"

Whatever method of travel you undertake always ensure that your equipment is handled with care on the journey, and carry it in a waterproof bag.

If you have mobility problems, or require help to carry your equipment, make advance arrangements for assistance at airports and railway stations. Get this organised when planning your journey.

Check ahead to make sure your accommodation is suitably located if you cannot manage stairs. For UK accessible holiday accommodation see **Appendix II Contacts List**

Remember to take extra care of your skin when you're out in the sun. Ensure you have access to suitable sun protection products when you're travelling to hot or sunny climates. **See Chapter 4 Skincare**

Anything else I should take with my ventilator?

In case of accidental damage to your mask you could take a spare one, and it's a good idea to take a fuse for the electrical plug. Don't forget spare filters, your chin strap if you use one, and any special cream or dressings which you use to protect your facial skin (and sun protection products if needed, as mentioned above).

It is always advisable to take an extension power cable. Unless you are familiar with the room in which you will be sleeping, you cannot be sure that there will be a bedside electric power point for you to use. If the only available socket is far from the bed, and the bed is too heavy to move, then you will need the extension cable.

You might also like to take a note of your ventilator's settings, along with the relevant telephone number to contact should your machine get lost or damaged.

When planning a journey abroad check that your equipment's voltage will be suitable. Some ventilators have adjustable voltage which enables them to be used in other countries.

> *The voltage on my CPAP is universal, so it's not a problem when I travel with it.*

If yours is not adjustable it may be possible to get suitable equipment on loan from your hospital. Check whether you'll need to take a plug adapter for the power socket.

My condition got worse when I went to Aviemore in Scotland

Respiratory and lung problems can be adversely affected by changes in altitude, for example in the Scottish Highlands where air pressure is lower. Blood oxygen levels fall at high altitudes. This could affect someone who already has a lower than normal blood oxygen level, leading to symptoms such as increased breathlessness, poor muscle tone and headaches. Some people are more affected than others.

> *In Scotland I get affected by shortness of breath and I tire very easily, but I know of someone who regularly visits the Highlands and hasn't had any problems.*

On some machines the settings can be changed to compensate for higher or lower altitudes. Check your instruction manual, or ask your hospital unit.

Should I ask my Doctor about air travel?

Reduced air pressure on board aircraft could affect you. If you have any medical problems, or have had previous difficulties when travelling, it's best to check with your Doctor before your journey.

> *I have travelled to many places in Spain and Greece with my BIPAP. I'm usually OK when flying. I just experience the odd headache sometimes, but nothing serious.*

Because air is re-circulated inside aircraft cabins it has a higher than normal level of carbon dioxide, and oxygen levels are typically lower than the normal atmosphere. For patients with a breathing disorder some hospitals will offer a Flight Assessment Test to find out whether air travel is likely to be a problem. The judicious use of oxygen on board the plane may be prescribed, if needed.

If you do require oxygen you must arrange it with the airline well in advance. There may be a charge for this. The British Lung Foundation help-line has information on the oxygen policies of major airlines. See **Appendix II Contacts List**

Incidentally, modern train carriages have sealed windows which cannot open and, as in an aircraft, the air is re-circulated. On a long journey there may be a similar possibility of lower oxygen and higher carbon dioxide levels in the ambient air.

Will I be able to get travel insurance?

Insurance policies often exclude pre-existing medical conditions, so you need to check this and make sure you are fully covered. Some insurance companies will not cover you at all, so you'll need to shop around.

> *I found a company which specialises in travel insurance for people with pre-existing medical conditions. There is a screening process, and although it is expensive, it is*

> *necessary to have adequate insurance when travelling.
> I had hoped to go to the USA one day, but sadly I
> have found that I couldn't even get a quote from
> some companies as I am considered high risk, and if
> hospitalised in the States it could be very expensive.*

Insurance may prove to be expensive, but it's risky to travel without sufficient cover for yourself and the equipment.

> *I have travelled to the USA with my Nippy ventilator.
> I didn't mention my medical condition because of the
> very high insurance premium, but it was not really a
> wise thing to do. I don't travel abroad now.*

Some Travel Insurance companies specialise in providing cover for travellers with medical conditions and disabilities, and do offer insurance cover for people who use NIV. See **Appendix II Contacts List**

Do I need to carry a letter from my Doctor?

The Insurance Company and/or the Airline may require a letter from your Doctor or Hospital Consultant detailing your condition and equipment, and stating that you are fit to travel. You should carry a copy of this in your hand luggage.

> *I always take a letter from my Consultant detailing my
> medical condition and explaining my need to use the
> BIPAP machine. I also place a copy inside the lid of my
> ventilator.*

Travellers planning to take any medication with them should check with the embassy of the country to which they will be travelling, to ensure that their drugs are not considered to be illegal narcotics there. Even over-the-counter drugs such as codeine may be prohibited in some countries. Drugs offences can carry heavy penalties, and ignorance of the law will not be a defence. Do not risk travelling with any prohibited substances; check for any regulations which may apply to your prescribed medications.

Ask your Doctor to give you a letter listing all the medications that you need to take with you, detailing the condition for which they are prescribed and the exact dosage that you need.

It is recommended that you have any medical letters translated into the language of the country to which you are travelling. Free translation services are available on the internet.

Hand luggage or baggage hold?

When travelling by air keep essential medical items with you, don't put them into the baggage hold. If you use inhalers carry them in your hand luggage along with your medications.

As for your ventilator, it would be very difficult for you if it gets lost or damaged on the journey. This is too big a risk for something so essential; therefore take it as hand luggage. Make sure that this is agreed in advance with the Airline and, as mentioned above, always take letters to cover it.

There could be hold-ups at Passport Control, as Security personnel may raise questions about letting your equipment, medication or oxygen cylinders through. Again this is something you should enquire about in advance: and remember to have your medical letters with you, so you can produce them when asked.

I always take my ventilator as hand-luggage, in a strong clear see-through PVC bag so the security people can see it.

In Brief

- ◆ Talk to your Doctor before making travel arrangements if you are going abroad, especially if you plan to go by air
- ◆ Make sure to take essential spares and all your equipment accessories when travelling
- ◆ Protect the equipment from damage and moisture en route
- ◆ If at all possible take your ventilator as hand luggage, as it may get damaged if it's put in with the suitcases
- ◆ Changes in altitude may affect some people with respiratory difficulties

- You may be affected by poor air quality on board aircraft - Flight Assessment Tests are available at some hospitals
- If oxygen is needed on the flight make sure your arrangements for it are in place before you travel
- Some Travel Insurance companies do offer cover for people with medical conditions but you may have to shop around
- If travelling abroad, plan well ahead and ensure you have all the paperwork and permissions needed to travel with your equipment
- Carry Doctor's or Consultant's letters about your equipment, medication and medical condition. Have your documents translated into the appropriate language

Part 3
TAKING CARE OF RELATIONSHIPS & FEELINGS

CHAPTER 7

Your Emotions & You

When they brought the machine to me, and said I would always need it, I was appalled.

Marion Mason

If you mention 'assisted ventilation' or 'mechanical respiratory support' many people will picture a very ill and debilitated bed-bound patient, being nursed in a high-tech Intensive Care Unit, perhaps lying in an iron lung.

Modern medical advances mean that patients no longer have to be restricted to iron lungs or long-term hospital care, but they can receive the respiratory support they need in their own homes. Their life expectancy will be extended, their quality of life will be improved, and in no way will their lives resemble that bleak vision described above. It is apparent that many people, both old and young, pursue active, motivated and productive lives while receiving mechanical ventilation at home.

At work I used to be so tired that I would fall asleep in the toilet, and I had trouble when taking dictation. When I got my ventilator it was a great relief to me. I noticed the difference straight away and was able to return to work.

It's all a bit daunting at the moment

For some people, using NIV will amount to not much more than an inconvenience or a slight adjustment to their daily routine. Others can find that their state of health now imposes some restrictions on them and they may lose the ability to do some of the things they'd like to do. It's natural that some patients will feel more vulnerable at first, and their self-esteem may be affected by this. But as their health improves they will begin to come to terms with the situation. Using NIV does not mean that you no longer 'have a life'.

> *In my experience the NIV made a huge difference to my life, but it was a good difference. For the first time in years I wasn't tired and breathless. I slept well, had renewed energy, and was able to embark on new intellectual challenges, so much so that, at the age of 50, I became a mature Degree Student.*

The improvements which the equipment and therapy brings to your health and energy levels will help to build your confidence in the treatment. Once you have become accustomed to using your medical equipment, and are feeling more experienced in managing this aspect of your health care, you will soon become quite blasé about the whole business. You'll find it easier to deal with those little day-to-day problems, and will look for creative solutions to coping with your changed circumstances.

This will reflect on the way people see you – as a confident, happy person, who stays well with the aid of a little bit of modern technological magic.

> *It was amazing how well I started to feel once I began using a ventilator, and I was very pleased. What pleased me less, however, was the fact that my Nippy was a large black box beside the bed, and I thought it looked rather out of place with the decor in my bedroom. It did depress me a bit. I tried draping a cloth over it when it wasn't being used, but that just looked silly. Then I had a brainwave – I took three jewellery boxes of varying sizes, and piled them up on top of the Nippy in a pyramid, with the smallest on top. It made my Nippy look like it was just part of an attractive display of boxes. Of course, I ALWAYS REMOVED those jewellery boxes before using the machine! More recently I was changed to the newer Nippy 3 which is much smaller and neater. It looks less obtrusive than the old one, so I don't need to disguise it, and the jewellery boxes have been put away.*

It's a very good idea to get into the habit of monitoring, and being aware of, your own state of health. After all, it's your body so you are the expert on how it is feeling and performing. Responsibility for your health care is first of all up to you. Look after your day-to-day health, be alert to feelings of tiredness, and pay attention to any unusual changes or discomfort. Keep yourself informed, do your best to have a healthy lifestyle, and make the most of your new lease of life.

> *My NIV definitely improved my health. I put on a bit of much-needed weight, my circulation improved, and I got fewer colds and chest infections. Now it is an accepted part of my life.*

See **Chapter 5 General Health Issues**, **Chapter 13 Diet & Nutrition**, **Chapter 14 Smoking**, and **Chapter 15 Exercise**

Friends have noticed my low self-esteem

Low self-esteem can be reflected unconsciously in your body language or tone of voice, and other people will pick up on this. Feeling angry or resentful, or blaming your 'bad luck', can only have a destructive action on your self-esteem, and friends may come to regard you as a negative person who should be avoided. See **Chapter 10 Dealing with the Feelings** for dealing with anxiety and negative feelings.

Dwelling on any negative aspects of NIV is not constructive. If you are having a problem, be pro-active and deal with it or ask for advice. Don't say you can't be bothered – take action!

Negativity can have a depressing effect on your general well-being, so try to focus instead on the many positive points of your NIV therapy.

> *I feel really lucky that my condition was diagnosed in time, and that the treatment is so easy to deal with. There's been no operations, drugs or injections, just my little night-time mechanical 'friend' that helps me sleep soundly throughout the night.*

If you do feel some sense of loss at first, developing a positive attitude will help you to feel that you are back in control of your life, no longer just a passive patient but someone who gets on with planning - and living - life again.

> *When I was told I needed a 'machine' I was very upset, and started to sob. I remember asking the doctor how long I would need to use it, and when she told me, "Forever," I felt so alone and sad, and couldn't stop crying. It came as such a shock – I was only 28 years old, had been married for just five years, my daughter was only two, and I needed a ventilator for the rest of my life!! I kept thinking I would not be able to be a proper Mummy and wife; I felt very worried that I would die young and that my daughter would have no Mummy. Well, how wrong was I? When I began to use my BIPAP at home it did take a while to get accustomed to it, but I am a pretty determined person, and I did get used to it. I am very lucky to have a good husband, and I got over the embarrassment of lying beside him, with the mask and headgear on. Now, after 14 years, it comes as second nature to me.*

I can't do all the things I used to

Most of us will eventually come to the realisation that as we get older some activities become harder, but disability or ill-health can also place restrictions on our life-style choices.

As a user of NIV, you may not always be able to do what you used to, and you need to help yourself come to terms with this. If you recognise your limits, and think of ways you can adapt, you will find out what you are able to do or you'll discover new methods of doing things, within your capabilities.

For example, if you enjoy gardening perhaps you are no longer able to tackle the heavier jobs. Light gardening tasks may be fine, and you can make adjustments to help you, such as using long-handled tools and having raised flower beds or planters, so that you don't have to bend over.

> *I like to potter in the garden when the weather is nice, even if it's just brushing up leaves.*

Don't be tempted to overdo things but learn to pace yourself, to avoid getting tired and out of breath. Have short periods of activity, with rest breaks in between. This way you will be able to continue with an activity which you enjoy (and in the case of gardening you'll continue to get the benefit of exercise and fresh air).

I think I'll try a new hobby now

Many people who start assisted ventilation therapy will find that life goes on much as before. There will be just a few adjustments, like re-arranging your bedroom, and organising arrangements to take your equipment with you when you travel.

But for those who have been quite ill, or who now have an impaired energy level, bigger adjustments may be needed. It's important to discover ways in which you can continue to have an enjoyable and active life. New hobbies and a good social network can help to avoid boredom and feelings of depression.

The British Lung Foundation advises that learning to live with a disability or medical condition can be a trigger for depression. This can make you feel like doing fewer activities or having fewer interests, which could then add to your depression. You may have been an active person and now can't do all the things you once enjoyed.

I am disappointed that I can no longer go camping. I used to enjoy my rural camping holidays, so I tried to find some other way to get enjoyment from the countryside. I decided to try my hand at watercolour painting, something I've always fancied but never got round to, and started going to local classes. These days I can still get pleasure from the countryside, but now I set up my easel in a suitable spot and get out my paints. It's great that passing walkers will stop for a friendly chat, and I also get the company of the birds and animals which come so close while I'm sitting there quietly painting.

If your previous hobbies prove too strenuous now, or you have extra spare time and are looking for something else to get involved with, you might consider taking this opportunity to pursue a new interest. Perhaps you'll try something which you've always been attracted to, but have never had the chance to do.

> *Despite my medical problems, I am a valued member of my local amateur dramatics group. I help the front-of-house team by taking tickets on the door, selling programmes and making the tea, etc. Whilst I can't take a singing or dancing role, I enjoy playing minor parts, when the opportunity arises.*

There's plenty to choose from - photography, cookery classes, a first-aid course, pottery-making, Open University, vintage car clubs, amateur pantomime groups, church activities, the local school committee, to name but a few. Perhaps you could become a volunteer for a Charity group. Your personal knowledge of living with a health condition could prove invaluable to such organisations.

> *I am on an Access Forum of eight people, helping with the access arrangements for places of historical interest. Everyone on the forum has disabilities so if one of us can't attend because of illness, the others understand.*

See also **Chapter 15 Exercise** for other activity suggestions.

I don't like being dependent on a machine

As mentioned at the beginning of this chapter, the stereotypical picture of a ventilator user can be hard to shake off, and no-one wants to identify with that. As you become stronger again, both mentally and physically, you will be able to dismiss that image as being irrelevant to your own life. You'll cease to regard your machine as a restriction, and instead view it as an aid to a healthy life.

> *A glamorous woman once told me that she would hate to be machine-dependent, and it really upset me at the time. Thinking back, I realise that such a response isn't unexpected. After all, none of us wants it, but when it happens to us we accept it, because our well-being is at stake.*

Many people depend on help, sometimes permanently, at various times in their lives – a plaster for a broken leg, a guide-dog for assistance, reading spectacles, a hearing-aid – and because all these are so common, they have become quite unremarkable. As more and more patients are prescribed NIV therapy, this also will become commonplace and unremarkable.

Let's face it, able-bodied people depend every day on all kinds of gadgets in the home, at work, on the land, and they can still kid themselves that they do it all by themselves!

Where else can I get advice & support?

This book can help to answer some of your concerns, but ideally you would chat to someone who is in the same position as yourself, so they could give you the benefit of their experience. If you don't know such a person, you may feel quite isolated.

> *I think new users, particularly if they are young, would benefit from contact with experienced users like myself. Many people seem to think that going onto ventilator support is the 'end of the road', but for me it was a new beginning. I knew that without my ventilator I would not have survived. It has enabled me to live an exceptionally active life.*

The support of your family and friends is, of course, important. However they may not understand the full effects of your condition, or they could find it hard to talk about.

> *My mother wanted to take all the family to a holiday camp, and said she'd book a large family chalet so we could all stay together. I tried to explain that I would need to be in separate accommodation because the others were not used to the sound of my equipment and it would disturb them. Mum just wouldn't accept that, and insisted that we must be together in one chalet, one big happy family. So I didn't go.*

Fortunately, through Support Groups, Charitable organisations, helplines and on-line forums, you can get advice about respiratory conditions, Sleep Apnoea and disabilities. You can also find out about local or national group meetings.

> *I do feel that you have to deal not only with the physical and medical issues, when trying to adjust to life with the ventilator, but also the different emotions that go along with it.*

Being in touch with others who have been through similar experiences can give reassurance that you too will be able to deal with your condition, and will help you build a supportive network of friends.

For example, The British Lung Foundation has a telephone helpline, and their website offers a great deal of relevant information for patients and their families. They have a nationwide network of social groups, called Breathe Easy. See **Appendix II Contacts List**, and **Chapter 8 Family, Friends & Work**

In Brief

- ◆ NIV need not stop you having a full and productive life
- ◆ It's natural to feel rather overwhelmed at first, but these feelings will pass
- ◆ If your favourite activities are now restricted, adapt the way you do them, or take up new interests and hobbies
- ◆ NIV is an aid to a healthy life, not a bar
- ◆ You are not alone: support and advice is available from many sources
- ◆ Your Physician can help if you are suffering from depression

CHAPTER 8

Family, Friends and Work

I don't think people really understand unless they have a similar condition. They seem to think it's like when they are a bit puffed after walking quickly, but it's not like that at all.

BIPAP user

Becoming a user of NIV can sometimes involve adjustments to your personal life and activities, and you'll need to learn how to deal with these changes. Adjustments of some kind may also be needed by your immediate family and friends. Strangely enough, the person who can help them best will be you! In the previous chapter we touched upon the ways your changed circumstances can impact upon family and friends. Even though the family wants to support you, they may also need encouragement and support. Sometimes we forget that they might be hurting and fearful too. Is your partner frightened they will not be able to cope, or that your intimate life together will be damaged? Do your friends understand that some activities may not be as easy for you now?

What about your children? Do you worry about their reaction to seeing your mask and machine – will they be frightened?

I don't want to scare my children

When you have children, especially little ones, you may worry that they will be upset when they see you wearing the mask. Only you can know how best to approach the subject with your own child, but a little preparation can be a great help, and treating the subject in a matter-of-fact way will prevent it from becoming a scary thing.

The picture book **'A Monkey, a Mouse and a CPAP Machine'** has been written for this purpose. This early reader/bedtime story book tells the story of Rufus the Chatty Chimp, who shows us around his home. He has lots of useful gadgets and equipment to help him in various ways, including his CPAP machine which helps him to sleep soundly at night. For availability see **Appendix II Contacts List**.

Together, you and your children can look at the book, and talk about how each gadget helps us. Bring up the subject of your own respiratory equipment, without any undue emphasis. You'll be able to say what the mask is, and how it helps you to keep well and happy at home. Perhaps you can discuss other people your family knows who also use medical aids – "Billy's Daddy has his leg in plaster, Granny needs a walking stick, Sarah's Mummy uses a wheelchair, and I have my ventilator!"

Alternatively, you could put together a little scrapbook yourself, which you and your children can read together. Cut pictures of everyday household gadgets from magazines and catalogues, and stick them in your book – vacuum cleaner, toaster, table-lamp, and so on. Include a picture of your ventilator, taken from an illustrated leaflet or downloaded from the internet. If you can't find a suitable picture, make a simple sketch yourself.

> *I remember being worried what my daughter would think when she saw me with this 'thing' on my face. We decided to just say that it is Mummy's ventilator - It helps Mummy while she is sleeping, and hopefully it will help her stay well so she doesn't have to go back into hospital. She was only 2 years old and, thankfully, she accepted it. I did worry she would be afraid of the machine, the noise, or the mask, but she was fine. The fact she was OK probably helped me cope better, knowing that she was not upset.*

When the machine arrives, talk about it casually and satisfy your children's curiosity. Some people find it helpful to call the hose and mask their elephant's trunk, or jet-pilot's mask. However, this may not be wise as it could encourage a child to think your equipment is a plaything. Be sure to let them know it is not a toy, and should not be played with.

Incidentally, if you worry that the noise of your equipment will prevent you from hearing your child crying in the night, go back to using a Baby Monitor in their bedroom again. This will reassure you.

My family is taking it harder than me!

It is not surprising that family members might find it hard to adjust to the situation. It can be distressing when someone close is diagnosed with a health problem. If it is a long-term condition there may be fears about the future, and if the problem is not a well-known one then there could be fear of the unknown. When someone is ill there are many aspects which can have an impact on the family, whether practical, financial, or emotional.

Money worries can be a real burden, so it's important to ensure that you are getting all the welfare benefits to which you are entitled - employment and support allowances, or sickness and disability-related benefits. Some financial help may be available towards home adaptations. Your own Doctor's practice will probably be able to organise free transport for your appointments at the hospital if you are unable to arrange transport yourself. See **Appendix II Contacts List**, and "I'd like to return to work" in this chapter.

The majority of NIV users will find that the treatment enables them to continue leading an independent and satisfying life, but it is a natural human response to speculate on what the future might bring. Family members could have concerns about their possible future caring responsibilities, should you ever need help with personal care. Reassure them that if this situation does arise, you will be able to investigate the financial and practical help available to you and the family, such as benefit allowances for carers. Social Services may be able to provide respite care, and gadgets to assist in the kitchen or bathroom. See **Appendix II Contacts List** for organisations offering information, advice and support to carers.

Even though they're concerned about your well-being, some people do find it hard to deal with sickness, hospitals and medical matters. Perhaps they have a hospital phobia and can't cope with it, so they just try to block it out. Exercise a little patience with them, and hope that they will be encouraged by how well you, yourself, deal with your condition.

I don't talk much about my health. My mother doesn't want to know – when I mention the subject she always assumes I blame her that I was born with this condition.

No doubt your family and friends will be familiar with that stereotypical image of a very sick person on a ventilator which was described at the beginning of the previous chapter, and this can be very upsetting. When they are ready to talk you can raise the subject. Ask how they feel, how it affects them and what worries them. Then you can work out how to deal with the situation, and how to reassure them.

Talk together; work through their fears or worries; don't let your illness come between you. Over time they will notice the machine's beneficial effects on you. They'll see you become confident in managing the machine and your own health, and that old image of an 'invalid' will fade.

> *When my partner was prescribed the use of a CPAP I was really upset at first. To me, mechanically assisted ventilation means a seriously ill person who has severe problems, and I had mixed feelings about it. Soon after she started with the CPAP, I woke up one night to go to the bathroom. When I came back into the bedroom I panicked – she was lying there so still, quiet, and peaceful, that I thought, "Oh no - the machine has killed her!" Of course, when I got closer, I saw that she was, in fact, sleeping deeply and breathing well. It hit me then how bad she had previously been – always thrashing about at night, gasping, waking, trying to breathe and never getting enough sleep. Now I am so grateful that she has been given the means to live a full, healthy, happy and active life.*

It's important to understand that sometimes people want to offer their support but feel unsure of how to do so. They may find it hard to express their feelings in words. Maybe they worry that talking about it will upset you, so they think it's best to say nothing at all.

Allowing them to help you in small, practical ways will enable them to express their support in a tangible manner. Perhaps they could give you a lift somewhere, collect your shopping, push the vacuum cleaner round, or cook you a meal. Of course, you may be very independent and therefore reluctant to accept help despite your medical condition, but by allowing them to offer practical help you will assist them to adjust to your new situation and to show their support without words.

It's hard to make my friends understand

Here's the problem. We don't always want to elaborate about our condition – after all, there's nothing more boring than someone going on about their health. Unless we go into some detail, however, people just will not begin to appreciate the realities of the difficulties we sometimes encounter.

People could think that all patients on NIV support are affected in exactly the same way. So if they know a CPAP user who leads a perfectly active life, (apart from the night-time respiratory support), they might assume that similarly you are hardly affected. If our own Doctor doesn't fully understand our condition, it's certainly not going to be that easy for the rest of our social circle!

You have to judge just how much information you are prepared to share. Most likely you'll disclose more to your close friends than to casual acquaintances, so their degree of empathy will naturally differ.

This is not to say that you shouldn't speak up when you need to. If you have problems keeping up with a group of friends, let them know, and ask them to slow down. It's perhaps advisable to sort out social engagements in advance. For example, if you're out with a group of people, you could arrange for a friend to lag behind with you, should the need arise.

I don't spontaneously say, "Yes," when invited out, as I have to consider things such as whether there will be stairs, or lots of walking, whether people will be smoking etc. Also, I have to use oxygen and feel a little embarrassed when people who don't know about it see me using it. (Not all my work colleagues know.) I don't go anywhere without taking a small oxygen cylinder with me and I transport it in a shopping trolley as it's too heavy for me to carry.

I'd like to carry on at my job

In the UK, under the Disability Discrimination Act, employers have responsibilities to make 'reasonable adjustments' to the work-place or conditions of employment, in order to accommodate an employee's disabilities. These adjustments include allowing you to make a phased return to work, time off for medical treatments, providing practical aids and equipment, or delegating someone else to do the tasks which you are no longer able to easily do. Grants may be available to help your employer provide equipment to assist you at work. Employees may also be able to get financial help for expenses such as fares to work. See **Appendix II Contacts List**

> *My employer is sympathetic. I have a trolley to use so I don't have to carry anything, for instance to the photocopier, and someone will always push it for me. I have oxygen in the desk drawer, should I need it. The Building Services Manager is aware, in case of Fire Drill or Bomb Alert procedures, and someone is assigned to ensure I get out of the building in an emergency.*

Some companies have excellent employment procedures and manage this aspect very well. If you find that you are unable to continue your job under the same conditions as before, it's better to deal with the subject before returning to work. When you're off work for a while stay in regular touch with your employers, keep them informed, and try to keep up-to-date on your area of business.

Consult your senior Manager, or Human Resources Department, and explain any difficulties to them. They may be able to arrange for you to return to work on a part-time basis at first, or they might organise transport for you if you need it. Perhaps a simple change of duties will help, or re-location to another part of the building, for instance on the ground floor instead of upstairs.

Be prepared to fully explain how your condition affects you, and what you can and cannot do, but be up-beat about it and show willingness to work together, so that your employer is on your side. Of course, you may still come up against that old problem of your employer or Department Head not understanding the implications of your condition, and its possible impact on your sleep or day-time function. You may need to explain that things which are not a problem for them can be difficult for you - an overnight power-cut for example, or the common cold.

> *I had a cold and a blocked nose, so my breathing was affected and I didn't get any sleep because I couldn't*

> *use the mask. I phoned work in the morning to say I couldn't go in, but my boss was angry. He said, "I come into work even when I've got the 'flu, so a little cold is no excuse."*

Educating others can sometimes feel like a never-ending job! In the worst case scenario, if you feel you are being discriminated against, you may need to seek employment advice. See **Appendix II Contacts List**

> *Until about a year ago I was working. My boss wanted me to change my hours and do the night shift instead. I explained that I couldn't because of my medical condition, but she wasn't sympathetic, and made me leave. I didn't take it to an industrial tribunal although I'm sure I had a good case.*

If your job involves driving, you may need to provide proof that your sleep disorder condition is being effectively treated and controlled, to avoid having your driving licence withdrawn.

I'd like to meet people and make new friends who understand my situation

Throughout the UK the British Lung Foundation has a network of social groups known as the Breathe Easy Club. These local groups hold regular meetings where you can meet other people with lung conditions. Breathe Easy also welcomes the friends and families of patients. Each group and its programme is organised by its own committee. Activities may include demonstrations and talks by guest speakers, excursions, fund-raising events, lunches, quizzes, and 'Sitting Exercise' sessions.

> *I always thought that Breathe Easy was meant for 'old' people, but when I went along I found that there were members of all ages, and I do really enjoy the meetings.*

Find details of your nearest Breathe Easy group on the British Lung Foundation website, or phone their helpline. See **Appendix II Contacts List** for details of organisations and websites where you can find Pen-pals, Friendships, Dating. See also **Chapter 9 Dating & Relationships**

In Brief

- Be matter-of-fact about your machine, so that your children are not unduly upset or scared. If there's time, prepare them in advance
- Family members may be upset or worried about you. They need time to adjust too
- Ensure you receive all benefits to which you are entitled, including carer's benefits for someone looking after you
- It's up to you to decide how much information you want to share with friends. More information will give them a better understanding of difficulties you may have
- Employers may be able to make adjustments to help you return to work, and in some cases may have a legal obligation to do so
- Keep your employer fully informed of your progress, and make advance preparations with the Company if you plan to return to work
- A local support group would be a good place for making new friends

CHAPTER 9

Dating and Relationships

I've not been offered any advice at all on the subject of relationships. I could have done with some, but didn't know who to turn to. It's not something I could discuss with my GP as he never has any time and isn't sympathetic at all.

BIPAP user

In this chapter we discuss whether people's feelings about relationships and dating change, once they become NIV users. This subject is important to many of us, and yet it's something about which we seldom receive advice.

Doctors talk to us about our physical health and fitness, and they'll help us to use the equipment, but the subject of our personal lives is usually not mentioned. If truth be told, this lack of advice is more likely to be because of time constraints in the clinic and the priority of restoring you to physical health, rather than it being considered as unimportant. Embarrassment might be a factor too. It is probable that most healthcare professionals receive no specific training, even at a basic level, for this aspect of their patients' needs, and without knowledge upon which to draw they will be reluctant to offer advice or make suggestions.

For some people, coming to terms with a medical condition and all that it entails can be quite a blow to self-esteem and feelings of attractiveness. With nobody to help us talk it through, it's easy to get the impression that loving relationships are no longer considered to be important for 'people like us'. However, many people can demonstrate that NIV is not a bar to healthy and happy relationships, so long as you adopt a positive attitude, and do not regard yourself as having an insurmountable handicap.

I feel that there will never be anyone for me – one look at me and they will be miles away!!

If you are upset by your condition, you have to face up to the fact that these unwarranted feelings of shame could be a bigger social disability than the medical condition itself. Work at accepting yourself: if you don't love yourself, how can you expect someone else to? See **Chapter 10 Dealing with the Feelings**.

I want to start dating again, but I've lost confidence and feel unattractive

First of all, let's consider the positive effects of your NIV treatment. Now that you're using the machine you'll be feeling more confident about your health-care than before. You'll begin to notice changes. Perhaps you'll have more energy, an increased sex drive, a healthier glow to your skin, and reduced snoring problems. These sorts of improvements can make you much more attractive as a potential partner.

> *I went through a time when I was very self-conscious about being a Nippy user, even during the day when I wasn't actually using it! I'd think about it all the time, especially when I was out socially. I would become so uptight that I appeared nervous on dates, which turned them off. After a few bad dates, I found myself thinking "Maybe I need a break from the dating scene". So I'd go out with the intention of just having fun and being sociable – not to get a date or anything. Interestingly, when I did this, I stopped thinking about my ventilator and I was able to relax more. Strangely enough, when I stopped trying to get dates, I found it easier to talk to women, and as a result I did get some dates!*

Coming to terms with a medical condition or disability is the first step to feeling good about yourself. It is an essential part in the process of accepting yourself as you are, and in deciding how you intend to get on with living your life.

If you feel it would help to contact others in a similar situation see **Appendix II Contacts List** for relevant contact details. It is good to know that it's normal to have these feelings, that you are not the only one, and that things will improve.

Once you feel more confident in yourself it will be easier to talk about health matters with new friends and partners. Confidence is an extremely attractive trait. The easiest part of this is to make the most of how you look. Find time to take care of your looks, grooming and clothing. It will reap great benefits in the long run. People don't mind the small details (like your machine) when the overall package is attractive!

How do I tell my new partner about it?

If you're in a relationship and your partner really likes you they won't be put off by the machine. If they are, then you have to wonder if they are really the right one for you. As hard as it is to accept sometimes, the old saying holds true – "There are plenty more fish in the sea."

When the conversation came round to my CPAP I just said that it stops me snoring and helps me have a good night's rest. It might look a bit unusual, but it keeps me fit. My girlfriend said, "OK, that's good then," and didn't seem bothered. Once I stopped caring, or worrying about whether or not it would freak her out, my attitude changed, and because I didn't feel it was such a big deal, she didn't either.

Obviously you don't need to bring up the subject on a first date, but you don't have to hide it either, should the conversation turn to the subject of medical matters. If your date visits you at home and sees the equipment, just be very matter-of-fact and explain it in simple terms. If they appear curious, show them the machine and the mask. Perhaps pop the mask on, so that they can see what it looks like on you. If they seem uncomfortable, or express concerns, you can help them to overcome any feelings of fear, discomfort or nervousness. Reframing the way they think about it can give reassurance. Get them to agree that all the fun things you've enjoyed together so far didn't involve the machine, so why should it matter now? Say it with confidence – it's a valid point!

In this situation your attitude is very important. If you appear nervous or embarrassed about it then you might scare them away. Talk about it matter-of-factly and you'll come across as strong and secure in yourself. Don't apologise as though it were a character flaw. Perhaps a little humour could be helpful: you could say that you think of it as your jet pilot's mask which helps you fly to the Land of Nod!

You shouldn't automatically assume that someone will react badly to your ventilator. You'll sometimes be surprised by the way other people view it:-

> *When I met Diana, Princess of Wales, I was asked to demonstrate my ventilator. I donned the mask, and switched the machine on. The Princess was not at all fazed or shocked but just said, "My boys would love to see this. They'd want to borrow it, to play Darth Vader!"*

Hopefully, the subject of your health will have already been discussed by the time your new relationship progresses from being casual to something more serious. If not, now is the time!

In the long run, being open and honest will be less painful than lying. By hiding the facts you imply that your condition is something to be ashamed of, or secretive about, and this gives it far more prominence than it deserves. When your partner does eventually find out, they will start to wonder things like:

- Why you have tried to hide it from me?
- Is it such a horrendous thing?
- Do you think I am so shallow that I'm incapable of understanding?
- Don't you trust me?
- What else are you hiding?

I'm afraid my partner will be horrified

There is no point in trying to second-guess what someone will think, you are not a mind-reader. You have to give them the chance to let you know how they feel. If it really freaks them out, then that particular relationship seems likely to fail, so you may as well find out before you get too deeply involved.

These days, a growing number of people are using CPAP machines for Sleep Apnoea, and so it is quite likely that your partner already knows of someone who uses ventilatory support similar to yours. If so, the concept will not be totally unfamiliar to them, and they are less likely to have hang-ups about it. They will react positively, and be pleased that you are trying to take care of your health. Some women may view it as a form of vulnerability, and actually regard it as a loveable and attractive trait in their man! When someone is genuinely interested in you they really won't care about your machine.

Never be tempted to do without your machine. Not only would you miss out on restful sleep, but you may jeopardise your health and well-being. No partner, however gorgeous, is worth that risk: and what if you snore so loudly without the equipment that your partner will be afraid to ever again sleep in the same bed as you?

> *The first time I spent a night with my new girlfriend I was too nervous to tell her. Yes, unwise, I know. I tried to stay awake, or just nap all night, while she slept. Next day I was so tired and unwell that she asked me what was wrong, and I had to come clean. Boy! Was she angry! Angry that I thought she would dump me over something so important to my life, and angry that I had risked my health. "How do you think I'd have felt," she asked, "if I'd woken to find you unconscious - or worse?" I had to admit that I should never have made those assumptions about her, and should never have put her in that situation. Lucky for me, she forgave me!*

Won't the noise keep my partner awake?

Early types of ventilators, although suitable for home use, were usually quite large and noisy. The Monnal D had an external bellows which inflated and deflated beside the patient and some people found it hard to sleep with all that huffing and blowing beside them! The Cuirass, which needed a very large separate pump unit on the floor by the bed, was even noisier. Modern ventilator machines run very quietly, so most people quickly get accustomed to the gentle sound. It's rather like going to live close to the ocean - you'll notice the sound of the waves at first, but you soon learn to tune them out.

> *My husband was concerned at first, but he got used to my Monnal D within a few nights. In fact, whenever I had to go into hospital for my overnight Sleep Studies,*

> *he would complain that he couldn't get to sleep as it was too quiet. I told him to switch on the vacuum cleaner if it was that bad!*

The sound of a CPAP machine will seem slight in comparison to the loud snoring, choking or thrashing about in bed of a person with Sleep Apnoea. The patient's sleep quality will improve, as will that of their bed-partner.

Of course if your bed-partner is a light sleeper there may be a problem, especially at first. Some people have overcome this with the use of ear plugs. Others find that having soft music playing as they drift off to sleep will help to cover the sound of the machine. If vibrations in the tubing are a cause of disturbance they can be reduced by wrapping your hose, perhaps in bubble-wrap or fleecy fabric, or you could buy a specialised Hose Wrap. For suppliers see **Appendix II Contacts List**

> *The Technician at my Lung Function Clinic told me he'd once had a patient who was troubled by the noise of her machine. (This was back in the days when ventilators were big and noisy.) She had a special bedside cabinet made, and put her ventilator inside. There was a vent to allow air into the cabinet, and a hole in the cabinet's side for the hose to go through. She needed a longer hose, and the Technician was able to supply her with an extra long one. The noise of the machine was muffled considerably by being inside the cabinet. Later she was moved onto an updated, quieter model and no longer needed the special cabinet. Modern ventilators are much quieter, and will not need such drastic measures.*

Another source of noise can be from air leaking around the mask, and these leaks should be dealt with in order to reduce or eliminate them. See **Chapter 3 Using the Equipment** for helpful tips on dealing with air leaks. Damage and deterioration can cause leaks or noise, so check the mask and hose regularly for signs of wear and tear. See **Chapter 2 Care of Your Equipment**

If you do find the noise very difficult to cope with, it may be worth enquiring if there is a quieter machine suitable for you, and whether you could be assessed for switching to it.

Even though it may take a while, it is worth persevering before you decide that the only solution is to sleep apart from your partner.

Unfortunately, sleeping in separate rooms can sometimes lead to other problems for partners. For a start, they miss out on the closeness of lying together, and the opportunities it affords for holding and cuddling during the night. Intimate love can feel less spontaneous if it has to be planned, rather than if it follows on naturally from goodnight hugs and kisses. On the plus side, both partners will enjoy a good night's uninterrupted and restful sleep.

However, separate sleeping arrangements need not lead to a couple growing apart. Having to plan your intimate time means it's less likely to be taken for granted or get boring. You could find that scheduling your 'snuggling time' at an earlier hour actually suits you better, rather than last thing at night when you're feeling tired after a busy day. Making a 'date' with your partner, just as in the early days of your relationship, could actually rekindle those feelings of romance and excitement, and bring you closer.

What about our intimate moments?

There is a time for sleeping, and a time for other things. The ventilator is needed only while you sleep, not when you're snuggling. It will not prevent intimacy, though you won't be able to roll over for a kiss in the middle of the night.

If your partner likes to sleep with their arms around you it may restrict the breathing movements of your chest. In that case, the 'spooning' position may be more comfortable. It's possible that excess air from your tubing could blow onto your partner during the night. But you might think this is actually handy during hot summer nights - just like having your own little air conditioning system!

Bed-time allows you to wind-down, talk to each other, have your intimate time, cuddles and kisses, just the same as any other couple. Then as soon as either of you feels sleepy you can say goodnight, put on your mask, and go to sleep. The machine becomes just one part of your normal bed-time routine.

My boyfriend has been using a CPAP for several years now. When we are going to be spending the night together he'll bring his CPAP machine. It's not a problem for me, and I've actually got so used to the sound of the machine it soothes me to sleep fairly quickly after he turns it on.

As a woman, I do feel unattractive now

I was doing very well on my CPAP, and feeling so much better. But I wasn't sure how my new boyfriend would feel about me wearing that mask every night, so I didn't tell him, and when I spent the night with him I didn't use my machine. Not only did my day-time tiredness return, but he started to make little jokes about my snoring. That certainly didn't make me feel any better about myself and I became more self-conscious about my condition. Eventually I took the plunge and was honest with him. I found some relevant information about Sleep Apnoea on the internet, to help explain the condition to him. Once he knew the facts he was so sweet and understanding about it, and I felt foolish that I'd not been up-front right from the beginning.

In this sort of situation, if you haven't been open about the subject, problems arise when the relationship becomes deeper. You sleep together more frequently, or you move in together, and it's not easy to suddenly reveal your bedroom 'secret'. Perhaps you'll be tempted to stop using the machine entirely, which obviously would have significant consequences for your health. See 'How do I tell my new partner about it' earlier in this chapter.

I felt ugly with a mask on my face and my hair all flattened by the straps. I worried that my husband would stop loving me. He's good-looking and able-

> *bodied, and I thought he might look for someone else. I realise now that he still loves me, despite me using the ventilator and looking like something out of a horror movie.*

Yes, it may be somewhat unusual, but it is not horrible! Try to look at it this way – this is a health issue, and if a partner can't deal with it they are valuing their own feelings above your health. The question you should be asking yourself is not, "How do I look?" but rather, "How do I feel?"

It may not be true of everyone, but in general women are often more likely than men to be concerned about body image issues. We are all self-conscious at times but there's less pressure on men. Women are constantly bombarded by images of unblemished skin, lovely hair, and a perfect figure, all of which they are supposed to aspire to. Television, movies, and magazines tell women that they are unattractive unless they measure up to these ideals. Suddenly having to cope with using a ventilator can be a blow to self-esteem, and make it difficult to feel attractive and desirable.

> *I got very depressed, and thought I would never be able to attract a partner. When I joined the Outsiders Club* (see Appendix II Contacts List) *I was put in touch with someone who had the same condition. She talked to me and gave me lots of encouragement, and happily I later met my fiancé through the club.*

It's not difficult to understand why people could have feelings of embarrassment, unattractiveness and sexual inhibition, but it's important to deal with these feelings and not let them stop you from complying with the treatment. See **Chapter 10 Dealing with the Feelings**.

If you've been feeling exhausted and sick, with interest in sexual intimacy at a very low level, then the thought of using a CPAP or ventilator could seem like the final blow to your relationship with your partner. In your eyes the machine may seem like an unwanted intruder in the bedroom, and a barrier to improving your relationship.

In fact, your sleep disorder itself is probably a major factor in the loss of your libido, your decreased desire, and the difficulty in achieving orgasm. If your condition has also been disturbing your bed partner's sleep, then the difficulties have been compounded, because neither of you is really in the best frame of mind for intimate satisfaction.

Rejecting your machine is not the answer. This leads only to a worsening of the symptoms and could threaten your health. The continued use of your NIV equipment helps you to sleep and feel better, gives you more energy, and improves your day-time functioning. Both you and your partner will benefit from fewer sleep disturbances, and sexual interest for both can increase as a consequence. Your treatment can improve your relationship, not damage it.

> *To be honest, I've found that men my age (I'm a woman in my forties) are often quite accepting of my CPAP. I think maybe they're becoming more aware of health issues, and they are even starting to worry that they might be falling apart themselves!*

As discussed in this chapter, the use of your ventilator brings improvements to your health, and this can have a positive effect on your attractiveness. Think about it: which is more attractive – snoring so loudly that you keep your partner awake all night, or sleeping quietly with a mask on your face? Refreshing sleep brings you improved health, renewed vigour, and greater energy. All these are attractive characteristics.

The British Lung Foundation has a series of helpful information leaflets for people living with lung conditions, including 'Sex & Breathlessness'. See **Appendix II Contacts List** for BLF details. Other useful contacts are listed there under 'Friendships, Pen Pals, Dating, Relationship Advice'.

In Brief

- ◆ The machine helps you to regain your health, vitality and attractiveness
- ◆ You don't have to tell all and sundry about your NIV, but if you're getting serious about someone, it's time to tell
- ◆ Treat it as no big deal. It's just another interesting thing about you, not something to hide or be ashamed of
- ◆ Never be tempted to do without the machine for the sake of a relationship – this could endanger your health

- When someone cares about you the machine will not make any difference
- The machine is just one aspect of your life: you use it when you SLEEP, not otherwise, and it doesn't prevent intimacy

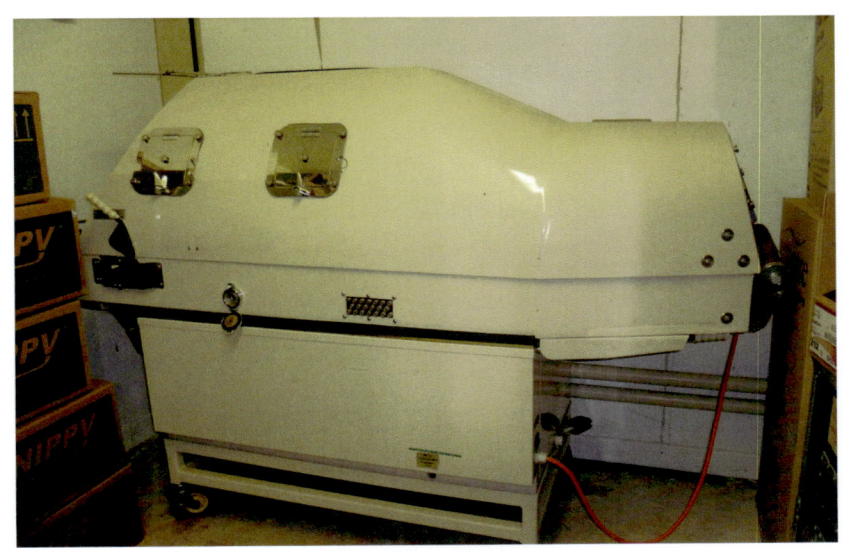

Iron Lung - Closed

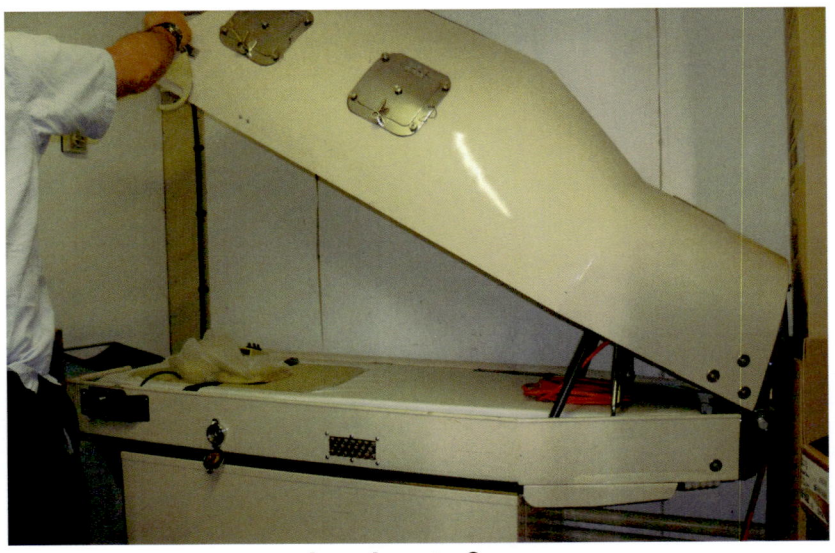

Iron Lung - Open

All photographs © Marion Mason except where otherwise stated

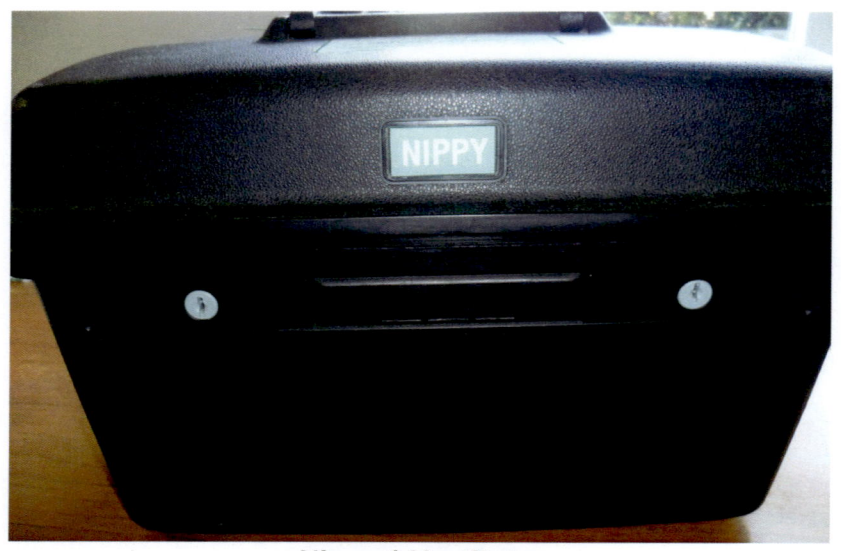

Nippy 1 Ventilator

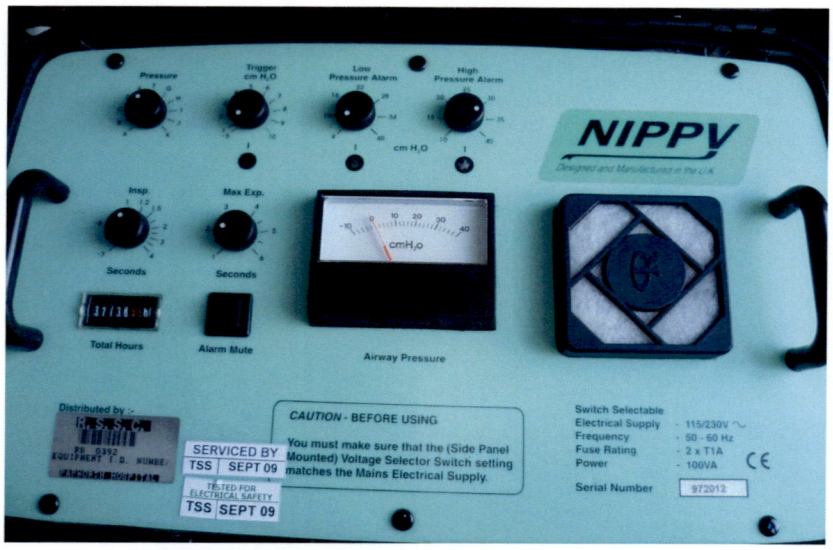

Nippy 1 interior showing square filter

94

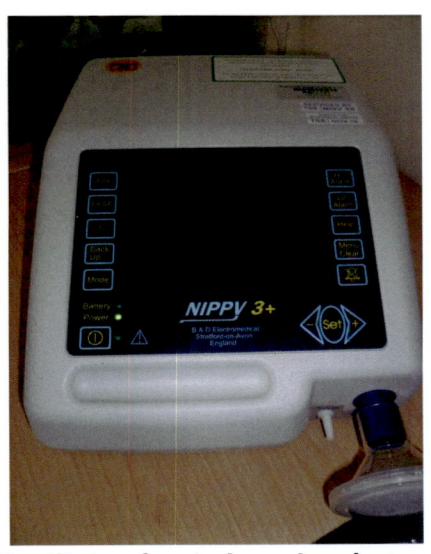

Nippy 3 Ventilator front view showing round filter

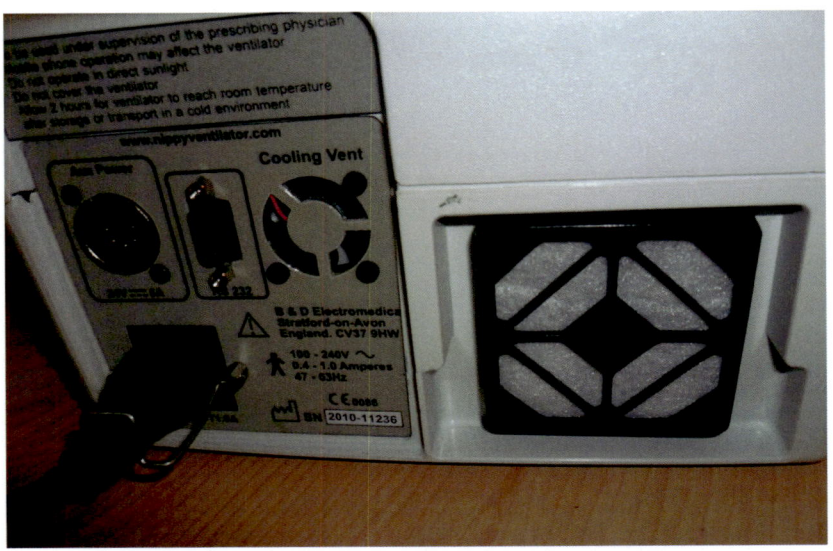

Nippy 3 Ventilator rear view showing square filter

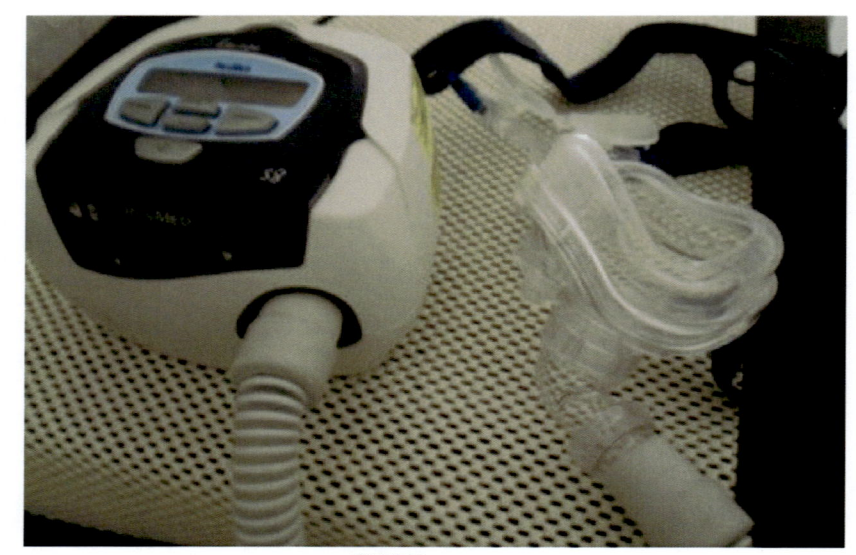

CPAP © J. Bilner

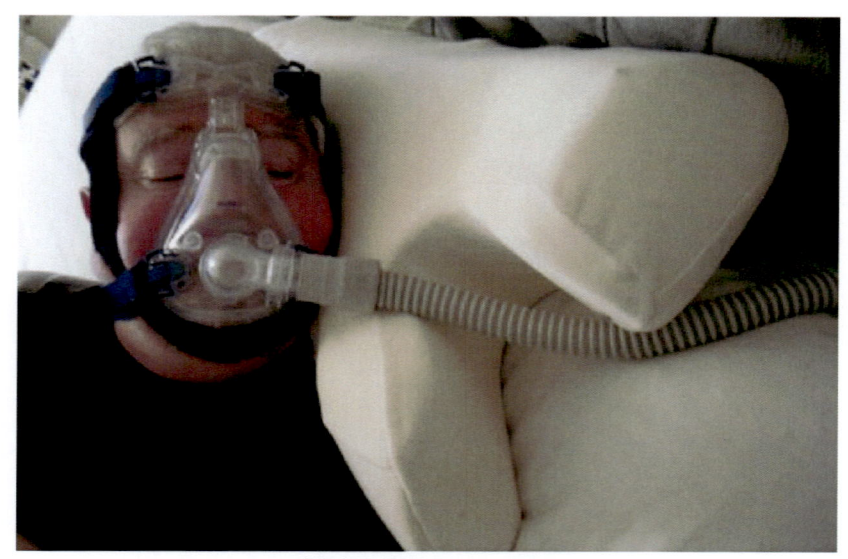

CPAP Pillow © J. Bilner

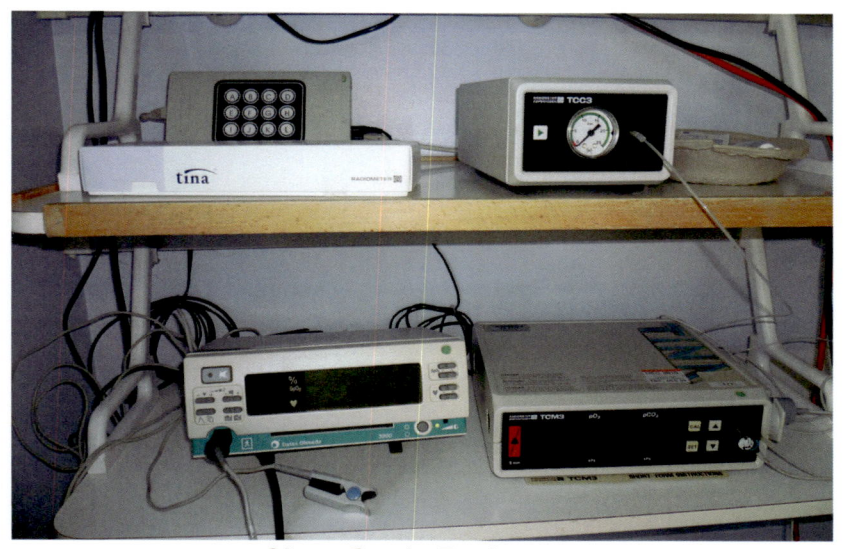

Sleep Study Equipment

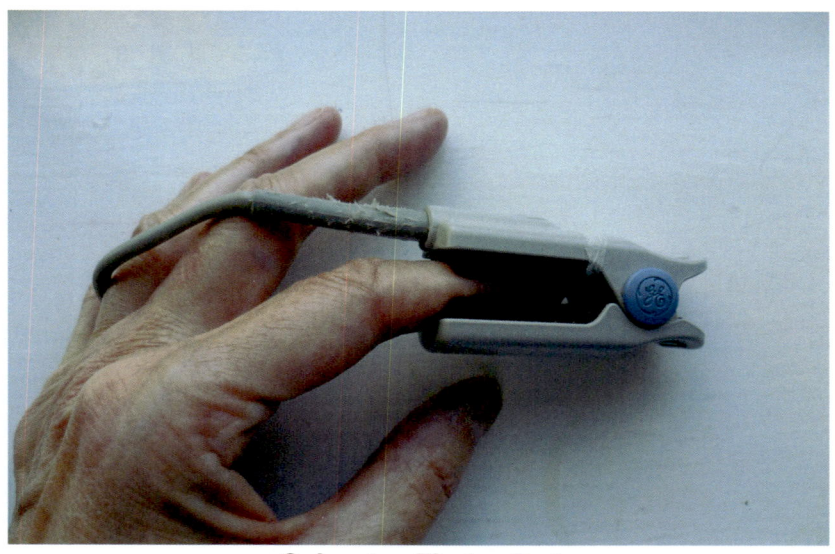

Oximeter Finger Peg

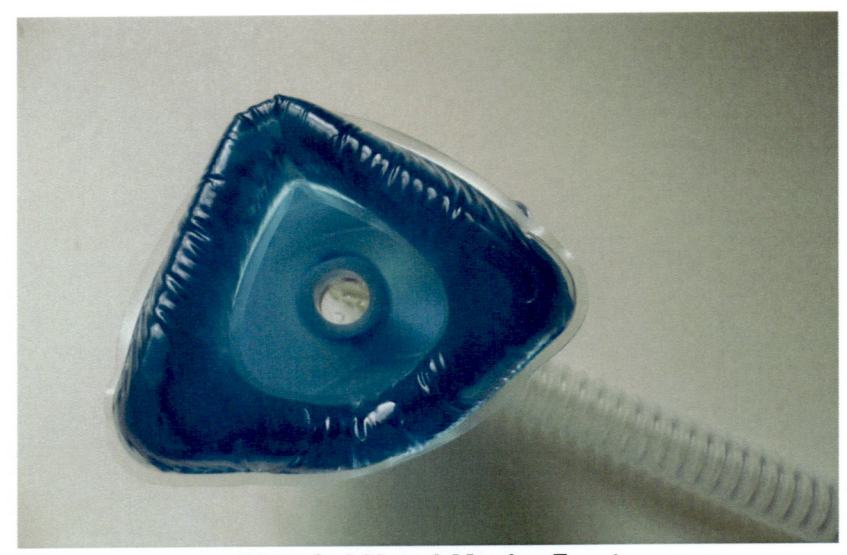

Blue Gel Nasal Mask - Front

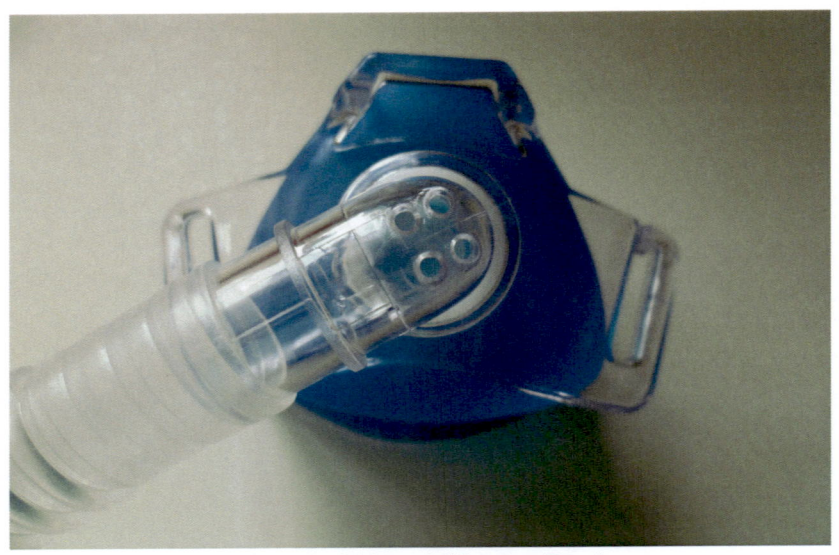

Blue Gel Nasal Mask - Back

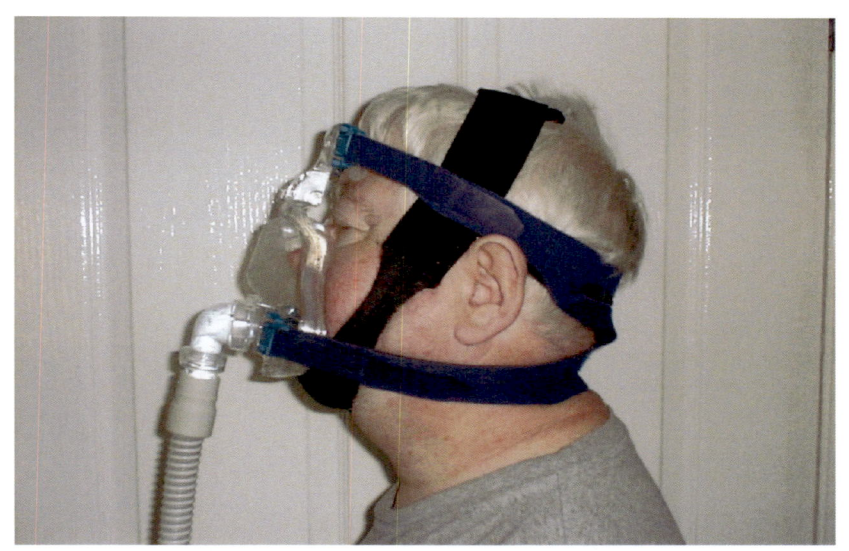

Full Face Mask and Secure Chin Strap

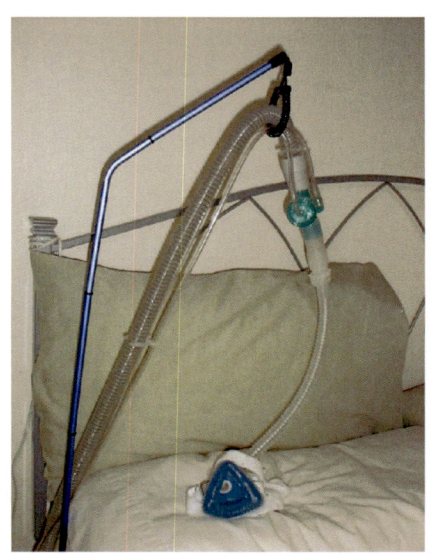

Hose Lift

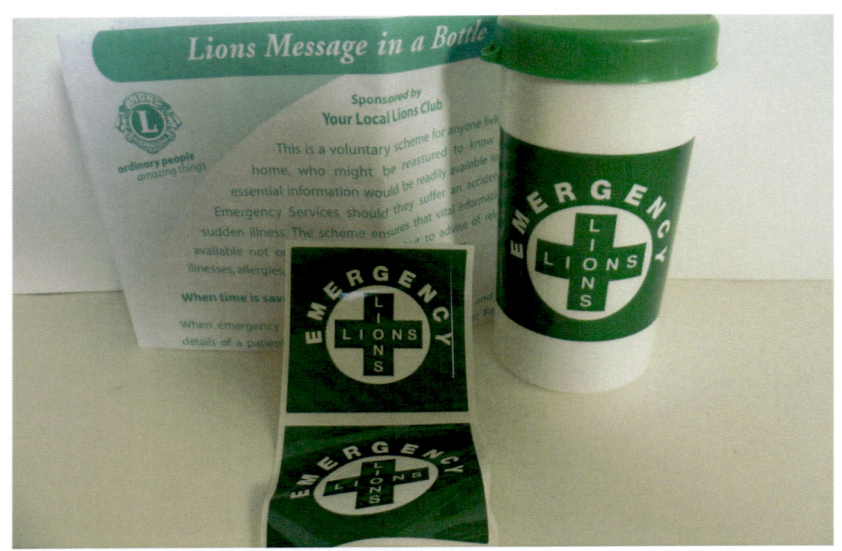

Message in a Bottle

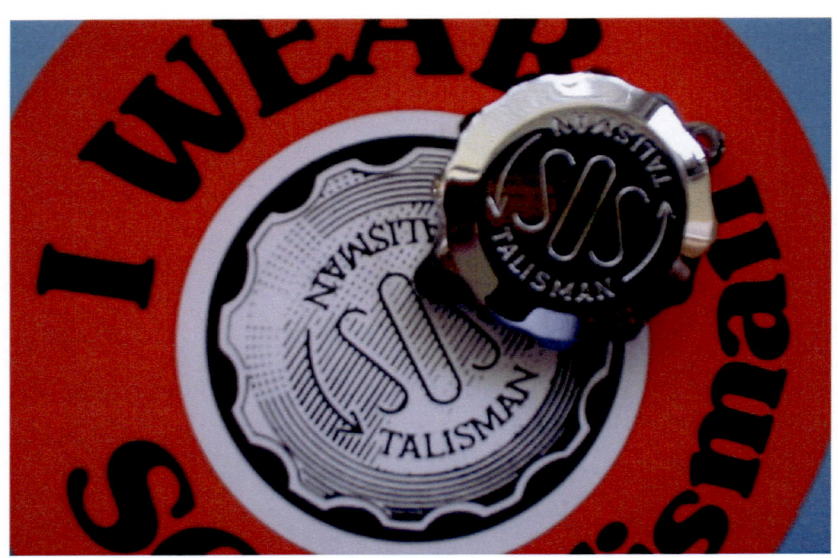

SOS Talisman

100

CHAPTER 10

Dealing with the Feelings

Life is like an arrow. You can hit the centre of the target, or you can shoot yourself in the foot!

Ted Nugent, Rock Musician

Steve Mason's ARROW Method   (ARRO)

If you have negative feelings or anxiety about using the NIV machine, here is a simple method to help you deal with the feelings. It is called the '**Arrow Method**' and is based on established principles from **Cognitive Behavioural Therapy**.

This method is intended to provide a user-friendly system for addressing negative emotions – whenever you need it.

There are four parts to the process:

- **A** - Accept
- **R** - Recognise
- **R** - Responsibility
- **O** – Overcome

Hence the name "**ARROW**"

Let's look at the stages in detail.

A: ACCEPT

Accept the feeling, whether it's fear, anxiety, embarrassment or frustration. Trying to ignore your feelings – bottling them up – is counterproductive. Instead, take time to sit down and acknowledge the feeling, and identify it.

R: RECOGNISE

The emotions and feelings which you experience are entirely normal.

Whenever we do something new or different we are bound to feel anxiety, trepidation, or anger.
Recognise and put a label on the feeling, and you will be in a far better place to deal with it.

At this stage, I use a 4-Step process - four simple questions that I ask myself. The purpose of these questions is to provide a framework for dealing with these emotions.

The questions are as follows −

- Why am I feeling this?
- What can I do about it?
- Do I want to get over this feeling?
- When do I want to get over it?

These questions help to identify the feelings in an objective way. Merely saying, "I'm depressed" will make you focus on the feeling, which will cause you to get even more depressed!

By going through this list of questions you are looking at the emotion from a third party perspective. It effectively gets you 'out of your head' and into a more positive, productive place.

The important thing is not to spend hours and hours thinking about the questions or trying to come up with answers. Don't make the mistake of over-analysing everything or assuming there is a correct or perfect answer.

Often our first impressions are the correct ones. You don't have to solve all your problems in one go; you can return to this process every time you need it.

Once you have done this you can proceed to the next step.

R: RESPONSIBILITY

By accepting responsibility for your feelings, and answering the four questions above, you have made a firm commitment to change. Many people have dreams and aspirations, but until concrete goals are set progress cannot be made. You cannot improve without some way of implementing that change, or without aiming for some sort of end result which can demonstrate that you've achieved it.

We can't always choose what happens to us. Some things will always be out of our control. However, we can choose how we respond to these things. We must accept that when we take responsibility for the way we deal with life, we empower ourselves.

For example, wishing you had the confidence to become a successful singer is an appealing fantasy. However, it is not a concrete goal. You have not taken responsibility for that goal.

The correct way would be to accept your goal, examine where you need to develop or improve, then set realistic targets to achieve it. If you have a good voice, but little confidence in front of crowds, then an appropriate plan of action would be to accept the problem, recognise the areas to improve upon, take responsibility for improving, and then go for it.

In our hypothetical example our aspiring singer would be best served by gaining performing experience. In that way, they can deal with the feelings and desensitise themselves to the more inappropriate parts of it.

A realistic goal would be 'To perform in front of a small, friendly crowd.' This could be as simple as regularly turning up at Karaoke nights with friends. Alternatively, joining a local theatre or amateur dramatics group would provide both support and experience. Having achieved success with this goal they can then move on to the next goal quickly and easily.

O: OVERCOME

First of all, remember that no feeling will last forever. Just because you feel nervous or angry now, doesn't mean you'll be feeling nervous or angry forever.

For example, at social events Steve, this author, has natural feelings of nervousness in meeting new people. However he knows that once the ice has been broken the feelings will go away, as he makes new friends.

Surrender to the moment. Never try to *force* yourself to overcome an emotion. That's a huge mistake. Whenever you're feeling shy, or uncomfortable, accept those feelings. Just doing this will often cause you to relax, and that negative feeling will naturally dissipate.

You now have a definite goal (or goals) in mind. You have accepted responsibility for your emotional state. With these tools you can work to overcome the feelings.

Many people have found that once they have started out on their plan everything seems to snowball in a positive way. You start paying more attention to your feelings, and deal with them appropriately. Likewise, you decide that while it is uncomfortable now to deal with your new partner's reaction to your machine, it is far better to be honest and discuss your feelings with that person sooner, rather than later. If you hide the fact that you use NIV, and betray the trust of your loved one, this will cause far more problems in the future than dealing with it now!

Other Helpful Tips

Get a mentor

If you're having trouble adapting to the machine, it's worth trying to get in contact with someone who has already gone through the same experience. They can provide motivation and help you through the hard parts. See **Appendix II Contacts List** for relevant organisations and forums.

Alternatively you may find it very inspiring to read about people who have overcome similar problems. To be honest, you may also find that you draw inspiration from people who don't have the same condition, but have still overcome the odds to get on with life.

For example, Simon Weston overcame horrific injuries that he received in the Falklands conflict. He successfully beat depression, and now is a tireless charity worker and devoted family man.

Many have been inspired by the story of athlete Lou Ferrigno, who was born with severe hearing problems. Ferrigno overcame an abusive upbringing by throwing himself into the sport of bodybuilding. Today Lou is regarded as one of the greatest ever athletes in that sport, alongside the likes of Arnold Schwarzenegger. He also achieved popular success as the star of the classic 1970s TV show 'The Incredible Hulk', where he starred with veteran character actor Bill Bixby.

Ferrigno has been quoted as saying "...if I hadn't lost some of my hearing I wouldn't be where I am now. It forced me to maximize my own potential. I had to be better than the average person in order to succeed."

There is sure to be someone, famous or not, who will inspire you.

Get educated

Often lack of knowledge causes fear or frustration. You may find that gaining more knowledge about Assisted Ventilation will help assuage your anxieties. The important part is to find positive information!

Only focus on information that benefits and inspires you. Constantly reading about the bad aspects of anything will cause you to develop a fixation on negative associations. What happens then is that you start to notice only the negative things. This makes things worse, which then makes you notice them again, and so on. It's a self-perpetuating cycle.

The part of the brain responsible for filtering in information from the outside world is called the Reticular Activating System, or RAS for short. The RAS filters through the millions of pieces of incoming information, allowing through only what is important or interesting to you at the present moment.

You will have noticed this in your life already. For example, if you have recently bought a red car, you will notice that you now seem to see red cars everywhere. Of course it's unlikely that there has been a sudden increase of red cars in your area; your RAS now knows that you're interested in red cars and makes you aware of them.

Some psychologists, therefore, will argue there is no such thing as 'reality'. Reality is actually only your own personal perception of the world and it depends entirely on what is important to you and what you are focusing on.

This means that you have to focus on something in order to get it, otherwise the information and the opportunities you need to get what you want will pass you by. Focus on negative things and that's what you'll notice.

In everyday terms – don't look for problems, unless you want to have even more of them!

Reward yourself

One of our correspondents used to find himself thinking about his machine a lot, and would even try to turn all conversations to health matters, just so he could 'vent' about his ventilator!

Luckily he realised this, and made a little game out of it. Whenever he started to think about the machine he would make a mental note of it, and then 'let it go'. He'd set himself small goals, like getting through the day without making a big deal about it or talking about it. Then he extended it to a few days - then a week. He'd reward himself with a treat when he hit the target he'd set. Eventually, he stopped caring and accepted the ventilator.

I just found that recognising how I was feeling, and then thinking, "Fair enough, mate, move on," worked for me. Sure, you have days when you find the whole thing a bit annoying, like when planning holidays, but the trick is to spot it, accept it, and move on. It's amazing how you can't think about it when you're busy doing something else, or while having a fun time with friends or family. Also it did help to learn that others felt the same way as me, and that I'm not unusual. We all tend to think we've got it worst, when we're down. The secret is to set little goals, and reward yourself when you achieve them.

Psychologists say that it takes about 30 days to accept a new habit and make it part of your everyday life. You may find it useful to keep a diary and tick off the days. If you have a slip-up one day, don't worry. Accept it and carry on. It's not what we do in the short term that matters – it's the long-term that counts!

Change your thinking

In **Cognitive Behavioural Therapy**, or **CBT** for short, there is the principle where you act 'as if' you have already overcome your problem. Then you note how you would feel if you truly considered the belief to be true.

Next you see yourself dealing with the situational challenges that arise, in the way you'd imagine would be correct if you had that new belief.

Finally you consider how other people would react, when they endorse your belief. You'll find that it works in a sort of circular way - you act in accordance with the new belief, and the positive results you get reinforce it, so it grows stronger, and so on!

If you want a quality, act as if you already had it. Try the 'as if' technique.

William James, American Psychologist & Philosopher

If you are interested in this method, then please ask your Doctor for the address of a good CBT therapist. Whilst CBT is meant to be a very simple, do-at-home therapy, you will find the guidance and experience of a qualified practitioner can help make the process more efficient, and it will work quicker.

Get a gimmick

This is obviously a very personal part of the process. What works for you may not work for others. If you have a highly personal – albeit effective – method, use it! Be careful of revealing it to friends though; they might find it amusing and their teasing could discourage you.

One young man found a very unusual way of overcoming his initial resistance to using NIV:

> *When I first started using the machine, I felt frustrated and anxious. I'd be filled with dread just putting on the mask at night. One day though, I was thinking that when it's switched on, the machine sounds a bit like Darth Vader breathing. So, when I settled down for the night I would just lie there, relax, and sort of pretend I was Darth Vader – "Luke, I am your father," sort of thing. It felt a bit silly, but laughing at myself doing a bad Darth Vader impression helped me to get over the feelings I was experiencing. And it worked. Even though I wouldn't necessarily tell my friends what I did, I found it did work for me. But if it works, use it, I say!*

Part 4
TAKING CARE OF YOURSELF

CHAPTER 11

Sensitivity to Indoor Pollution

...it's important to ensure that the air we breathe in our homes (or where we work) is as clear and unpolluted as possible

British Lung Foundation

If you are sensitive to chemicals, smoke or other pollutants it may be difficult to avoid them in the environment and in other people's houses, but there are steps you can take to reduce exposure in your own home.

I don't use air freshener sprays as these make my breathing worse. Perfumes and aftershaves are OK as long as they're not too strong.

General advice:

- ◆ Let fresh air into your home as often as possible. Open your windows for a while each day to replace the stale air and help eliminate condensation and moulds

- ◆ Warm-air central heating which works by circulating warmed air round the home will also waft dust particles around. Always keep the central heating grilles free from dust, and follow the manufacturer's cleaning and maintenance instructions

- ◆ Your ventilation machine draws in ambient air, i.e. air from your bedroom, and feeds it to your lungs under pressure. Nearby smells, dusts or chemicals can be drawn in too, and may not be completely eliminated by the filters, so it's important to avoid these pollutants as much as possible

- Check your machine's filters weekly and replace them if necessary. Dirty filters will not function efficiently. See **Chapter 2 Care of Your Equipment**.
- Always use household cleansers, aerosols, paints etc. in a well-ventilated area. Carefully follow the directions given on the label, and do not use different products together as the combination may produce unpleasant fumes

The strong smells from some perfumes and cleaning products give me a coughing fit – I have asthma.

- Vacuum-clean your upholstered furniture, curtains and drapes, and wipe window blinds
- Take care when vacuuming as it can disturb dust which then circulates in the air
- Groom your pets outside
- When dusting use a damp cloth or an electrostatic dusting cloth, so that dust is collected without being knocked into the air

Bathroom:

- Did you know that a fine mist of droplets is sprayed into the air if the toilet is flushed with the lid open? This spray contains traces of cleansing products as well as germs. It can circulate in the home, or settle on nearby surfaces, so remember to close the lid before flushing
- If the bathroom is close to your bedroom it may not be a good idea to put your cleanser products down the toilet last thing at night. The smell of these strong chemicals can linger in the air, and may reach your ventilator in the bedroom, especially if you've forgotten to close the toilet lid
- Carpet in the bathroom is unhygienic. It gets damp and cannot be easily cleaned. This encourages the growth of moulds and bacteria. Washable cotton mats are preferable as they can be kept clean and hygienic

Bedroom:

- Keep pets out of the bedroom and do not let them sleep on the bed
- Padded headboards get dusty so vacuum-clean them when you do the carpets
- The mattress should be vacuumed occasionally too
- Anti-allergy mattress protectors are available at bed-linen stores
- When decorating the bedroom make sure it is thoroughly aired before you resume sleeping there
- Examine your machine's filters regularly, and clean or replace them as required. See **Chapter 2 Care of Your Equipment**

Air Freshener Products:

- Household air freshener products are a common irritant
- Some room air-fresheners work by being plugged into a power point. These can emit a very pungent smell, whether or not the power is switched on. If you have one situated in, or close to, your bedroom it may affect you, even if it's switched off at night
- Avoid using air fresheners and spray polish in your car, as these will have a stronger effect within the enclosed confines of the vehicle
- Scented candles and joss-sticks may affect some people

Laundry:

- Perfumed fabric conditioners can cause problems for sensitive people. Some are formulated so that their odour is released not only when clothing is freshly laundered, but whenever the garment is rubbed while it is being worn. This is not ideal if you are sensitive
- Un-perfumed laundry detergents and fabric conditioners are available, and would be more suitable for sensitive skins and noses
- Pollen can settle on the fibres of clothing and linen, so if you are sensitive to it do not hang out your washing to dry on high pollen days

Tobacco and Smoke:

- People with a respiratory condition can find that tobacco smoke affects them very badly, especially in a confined space such as a vehicle

- If family members smoke they should be encouraged to smoke outside, not indoors

- Even if you restrict smoking to only one room of the house, the smoke can circulate and permeate the rest of your home, despite best intentions

- If you share your home with a smoker your machine's filters will need replacements more frequently. Check them weekly. The filters may not totally prevent fumes and chemical substances from passing through especially when the filters need to be replaced. (During the day you'll be breathing in any smoke in your home, without the benefit of filters.) See **Chapter 14 Smoking**, for tips on giving up, and **Chapter 2 Care of Your Equipment** for information about filters

Pets:

- Pet hairs, fur and feathers can be the cause of allergy for some people. Groom pets outside, and keep them off your bed

- If you have household pets it's important to regularly vacuum the carpets and soft furnishings, and to dust hard surfaces

- Animals are best kept away from your bedroom and equipment

Wooden and Vinyl floors:

- Many people prefer wooden floors or vinyl flooring, either because it fits their décor, or because they feel that carpeting can attract a build-up of dust

- Dust and pet hairs will settle and stick onto a carpet, where they stay until vacuumed off

- On a smooth floor the dust and hairs lay loosely on the surface, but if disturbed by air currents, or by someone walking past, they will be propelled into the air again

◆ It is important to keep smooth floors free of dust, and such flooring could require daily cleaning to eliminate dust and particles which settle on it. Wipe over frequently, to keep dust levels low

◆ It is, of course, also necessary to vacuum carpets regularly

In Brief

◆ Do your best to keep your home free from any pollutants that may affect you

◆ Don't neglect to check your ventilator's filters every week

◆ Your own Doctor can prescribe anti-histamine tablets, nasal sprays and other medications to treat allergies

◆ Consult your Doctor if you experience persistent allergic symptoms or sensitivities

◆ Seek medical advice without delay if an allergic reaction or sensitivity is making it difficult for you to use your ventilation equipment

◆ For further information on allergies, asthma and sensitivities see **Appendix II Contacts List**

CHAPTER 12

Health Information for Emergencies

In case of an accident... you may not be able to communicate to the emergency services. Many patients are transported to the hospital alone, without relatives or friends to discuss possible life saving medical history.

Medical Tags UK

Should I carry health information in case of a medical emergency?

It is possible that your hospital will issue you with a card for emergency situations, upon request. Alternatively you could write one yourself, and put it in your wallet or bag where it can easily be found.

I carry a card from the Polio Fellowship stating that I have Post-Polio Syndrome which causes breathing difficulties.

The Sleep Apnoea Trust offers a card for CPAP users. See **Appendix II Contacts List**

Instead of carrying a card, some people prefer to wear some kind of medical identification tag to bring attention to their medical needs. Emergency staff and personnel are trained to check for these information tags.

These items are also known as medical jewellery, drug allergy tags or emergency tags.

They are available in a range of attractive, stylish designs, colours and prices. There are bracelets, necklets, watches and dog tags. For sports wear there are bracelets with coloured canvas or elasticated straps, and for children there are attractive designs including butterflies, footballs and flowers.

Some of these pieces are engraved with essential medical information and contact details. Others incorporate a capsule containing a folded strip of paper on which you write your details.

When I go out clubbing, people often admire my rubber necklet with its metal pendant and ask where they can get one. They are so surprised when I say it's my Allertag ™

See **Appendix II Contacts List** for details of suppliers.
Other similar schemes can be found on the internet.

The Medical Tags Company

This company can supply a wide selection of medical identification jewellery, including the SOS Talisman items.

Medic-Alert

This is a charitable organisation. You register with them and they make a record of all your medical details. There is an annual fee, but this is sometimes subsidised, or free, for those on a low income or in receipt of certain benefits.

Once registered you purchase a bracelet or necklet to wear. This will be engraved with your vital medical information and a personal identification number, along with the telephone number of the Medic Alert 24 hour service.

In an emergency Medic-Alert can be contacted for the details of your medical history on their data-base. This service accepts reverse charge calls and can give information in over 100 languages, so that medical and emergency professionals can access your details from anywhere in the world.

SOS-Talisman

The SOS-Talisman company supplies bracelets and pendants with a water-proof capsule section in which to enclose a note of all your details.

With your purchase you receive a long, narrow strip of water resistant paper which folds neatly to slip inside the capsule. You have to fill in the details on the strip yourself. It would be advisable to use a permanent marker pen for this. There is no back-up as with Medic-Alert, and no further charge.

Key-ring fobs, car stickers, luggage tags and other items bearing the SOS logo are available. These help to show emergency services that you are wearing an SOS Talisman.

The Lions Club 'Message in a Bottle' scheme

Pack available free from some Pharmacies, Doctors' surgeries, Age UK, Police Stations, Housing Associations, Charity shops etc. Or contact your nearest Lions Club.

This UK scheme, sponsored by the Lions Club, ensures that vital information is available if you have a domestic accident, or are taken suddenly ill at home. You are supplied with a plastic bottle which has a lid and is clearly marked with a green cross. Inside are two Green Cross stickers and a form.

Complete the form with all your details including medical condition, medication and medical equipment, allergies and contact addresses. Place the completed form into the bottle, seal the lid, and place the bottle in your fridge in the door compartment, where it will be safe and can easily be found. Stick one of the Green Cross stickers on the outside of the fridge door, and the other inside your front door at eye level, (making sure it is not visible from outside).

If emergency services are called to your home the Green Cross stickers will immediately indicate that you have a 'Message in a Bottle', and they will know where to find it. Extra forms are available. A separate form should be completed for each member of the household.

The following simple idea can be used by anyone who carries a mobile/cell phone.

The I.C.E. System – This stands for 'In case of Emergency'

This concept was devised so that emergency services or medical staff can easily identify which telephone number on a person's mobile/cell phone belongs to their next-of-kin.

It's simple to take part - all you have to do is to store on your phone the telephone number of the person who should be contacted in an emergency, under the initials **ICE instead of their name.**

If you are taken ill, or involved in an accident, the emergency services will quickly be able to contact the right person by dialling the number you have stored as **ICE**. For more than one contact, name them **ICE 1, ICE 2** and so on.

Of course you should think about carrying standard forms of identification too. Remember that if your phone is secured by a PIN number this will block attempts by emergency personnel to access the information.

Important advice for NIV users

If you are admitted to hospital ensure that your Ventilator or CPAP is taken with you. When being transported by ambulance, tell the ambulance crew about your condition and equipment.

You might be admitted to a ward where the staff are not familiar with your equipment, or do not know how it works. Ask them to phone your specialist unit, if that is the case. Make sure your ventilator is set up and plugged into a power point, to enable you to use it without delay as soon as you need to.

For some ventilator users, oxygen may possibly be detrimental unless administered **through the ventilator.** Ask your Physician if this would apply to you and, if so, ensure you tell ambulance and hospital personnel. **It is essential to include this information in the emergency details you carry or wear.**

> *I carry a hospital note which says I mustn't be given more than 27% oxygen, and also states I should be taken to a hospital with a Lung Function Clinic.*

In Brief

- Take all your equipment and medication with you if you are admitted to hospital
- Make sure the hospital staff understand your condition and the use of the equipment
- Ask for your ventilator to be set up as soon as possible, in case you need it

Chapter 12: Health Information for Emergencies

- Carry some form of medical information in case of emergency
- Put all your medical details in a prominent place at home where they can easily be found
- Save important contact numbers onto your mobile phone under the name ICE

CHAPTER 13

Diet & Nutrition

A healthy, nutritious diet can help you look and feel your best, and is easier than you might think.

NHS UK

One of the keys to good health and managing your respiratory condition is to follow good dietary habits. Quality and content of your food is important, and there is a wealth of information widely available to help you. Magazines and TV shows often feature articles on cooking, nutrition and diet, although it's important to sift out the faddy celebrity-endorsed diet plans from the sound nutritional advice. There are plenty of good books and websites to cater for all tastes - vegetarian and vegan meals for example. Your Physician or Clinic will also be able to offer advice, and help you take a pro-active role in this aspect of your well-being.

Being overweight is a factor in health issues such as varicose veins, skin infections, aching joints, diabetes, raised blood pressure, osteoarthritis and depression. Extra weight means greater demands on heart and lungs. People using assisted ventilation may find that their breathing problems are increased if they gain weight, because their lungs struggle to cope with the extra body mass. Larger people have an increased risk of developing Obstructive Sleep Apnoea (OSA). Studies suggest that symptoms of OSA are generally worse for those who are overweight, but by losing excess pounds the degree of this breathing disorder can be reduced.

Similarly, being underweight can have health implications: lower energy levels, tiredness, muscle breakdown, anaemia, osteoporosis and a less effective immune system.

Small changes to the daily diet can make a big difference. This chapter covers useful tips for changing eating habits without using extreme methods, whether you are trying to lose or gain a few pounds. **Appendix II Contacts List** has details of useful organisations providing sound nutritional advice. See also **Chapter 15 Exercise**

Should I see my Doctor about my weight?

If you're worried about being over or under weight, or if you lose or gain weight quickly, consult your Physician. Tests will discover whether the cause is an underlying medical problem, such as a thyroid condition. Steroid treatment can be a cause of weight-gain, as well as contributing to sleepless nights, mood changes and increased feelings of hunger.

Your Doctor will prescribe medication, offer dietary guidelines, or refer you to a dietician, as appropriate.

I've tried lots of celebrity diets but they don't work

Let's be honest here - faddy and extreme 'diets' do not work. Celebrity-endorsed diets or other weird regimens usually involve an extremely restricted diet – perhaps only having cabbage soup, grapefruit or apples. Such a narrow range of food puts the body in danger of vitamin and mineral deficiencies, along with insufficient intake of protein. In any case it's hard to keep up such a diet for long, and you are very likely to give it up and go back to your old habits.

Extreme diets, vomiting, laxatives, purging, starvation and self-denial do not work and can seriously damage your health.

> *A friend of mine tried the 'cabbage soup' diet. She hated it, but it worked and she lost a lot of weight. To celebrate her weight loss she had double cheeseburger and chips at a fast-food outlet. She went straight back to her old eating habits and wondered why she put the weight back on again!*

Initially a very strict crash diet may help you to lose weight, but as soon as you return to your old eating patterns you'll regain the weight, sometimes more than you lost. Blaming the diet, saying it didn't work, and then trying yet another different scheme, just leads to 'yo-yo' dieting, which is not good for your health or your self-esteem.

Instead of quick-fix starvation diets, you should aim for a sustainable plan which you will be able to stick to all the time, not just for a week or two – a 'Diet for Life'. Stop counting calories. Instead, make a change in your long-term eating habits. It need not be a difficult process and doesn't mean you'll have to totally deny yourself all the things you like. Just have them in moderation, along with eating as healthily as you can.

Have realistic weight-loss expectations and aims. 'Slow-but-sure' is preferable to extremes, so aim for a modest weight loss per month, not a large amount. Lose too much too quickly and you run the risk of losing muscle instead of fat. Just cutting out one daily snack would make a difference. One chocolate biscuit per day can amount to several pounds over the space of 12 months! Reducing your alcohol intake will also reduce your calories.

I couldn't possibly give up chocolate

The problem with restricted diets is that they can encourage you to fixate or obsess about certain foods. If your food plan bans something you really like, you will want the 'forbidden' food. Then, when you do lose a little weight you'll be tempted to reward yourself with that forbidden food. It seems more sensible to have a small piece of chocolate now and again, rather than to deny yourself any chocolate at all, then give in to temptation and gobble up a whole bar!

Your 'diet for life' doesn't have to exclude your favourite foods entirely. Have just a small portion or try a healthier version. If you can't resist chips/fries, try thick oven-baked chips or wedges instead. Buy them frozen, or make them at home yourself, it's not difficult. Grill, steam, stir-fry or bake food rather than frying it. Fish is a good protein source, but avoid battered fish. Speciality breads are tasty without butter or spreads, and are a great accompaniment to salad or home-made soup.

As with many things moderation is the key, along with a sensible approach to food, and a healthy eating plan.

I don't eat unless I'm really hungry

This is not a good strategy for losing weight. If you are frequently hungry your body will go into starvation mode and retain fat reserves, using energy from muscle tissue instead. You'll keep the fat but lose muscle.

Another danger of letting yourself get extremely hungry is that the hunger will cause your brain to compensate by triggering the desire for high calorie, sugary, fatty foods. When you do eventually eat, you are more likely to want fattening foods, to eat more than you really need, and even to binge-eat.

Your aims should be: Never reach the stage where you are extremely hungry, and never eat so much that you feel stuffed. There's no need to starve yourself, but neither should you overeat.

Four small meals a day, rather than two large ones, will keep up your energy and blood-sugar levels all day, and prevent that feeling of extreme hunger. Perhaps you'd prefer three meals, with a couple of small, healthy snacks. Decide which eating pattern fits your personal daily routine and suits your needs, and incorporate the tips shown further on in this chapter.

I just can't face food first thing in the morning

It is said that breakfast is probably the most important meal of the day. As you haven't eaten since the previous evening your blood-sugar levels are low. If you skip breakfast, you'll probably feel too hungry later on, and will be more likely to start snacking, or to eat too much. See previous section.

> *My partner insisted we go out shopping very early, and we had no time for breakfast. After a couple of hours at the DIY & Garden Centre we were both flagging and hungry, so we stopped for Danish pastries and frothy coffee at the in-store Coffee Shop. Not a healthy choice!*

Some people really don't feel like eating first thing in the morning, but even something very simple such as a banana, a few sultanas, a yogurt or a slice of whole-grain toast will help to 'break your fast' and perk you up. It might even kick-start your appetite so that you do feel able to eat a bit of breakfast after all.

I often feel peckish

Sometimes thirst can be mistaken for hunger pangs and you actually need a drink, rather than something to eat. Try drinking a cup of tea or some water when you feel peckish, instead of reaching for a biscuit.

As an alternative to plain, cold water have hot water with a slice of fresh lemon. A little cranberry juice will add sweetness if needed. Try adding a piece of fresh ginger for extra flavour. Use a slice of orange instead of the lemon if you have a sensitive stomach.

After your drink, if you're still hungry, then have something to eat, but don't eat a packet of biscuits while the dinner is cooking!

What are the tips for a 'Diet for Life'?

I am overweight and am trying to lose a few pounds. I've cut down on chocolates and sweet things, but I'd appreciate some tips to help me.

Here are some suggestions which may be useful. Read through the list and see which ones could help you.

CUTTING DOWN ON SNACKS

- Don't eat just because you're bored. Go out and get some fresh air instead, or spend time on a hobby or book
- Don't snack or eat 'on the run'. Sit down to eat
- Cut out fizzy drinks / soda pops
- If you feel hungry maybe you just need a drink, so have some water or a cup of tea
- If you still feel hungry after your drink then have something to eat. Don't wait until you're feeling famished. Prepare a meal or have a healthy snack
- Finger-food is so convenient, but it's easy to over-eat. Eat with a fork where possible, and don't eat straight from a packet. If you dip into that large pack of potato chips or popcorn it's easy to eat more than you realise. Eat your portion from a small dish and put the packet away!
- If you're distracted by TV or a book while you're eating you could easily eat more than you need. Beware of cinema snacks – your 'bucket' of popcorn contains a lot of calories and you can easily plough your way through it without even noticing

I love jelly bean sweets so I'm easily tempted. I opened a packet, intending to have one or two while I played a computer game, but before I knew it I'd eaten the whole pack!

MEAL TIMES

- Use a smaller than usual plate or dish; your portion size will be smaller even though your plate is full, and you will be less likely to continue eating when you're full up
- Eat slowly and savour your food
- Stop eating when you feel full. You don't have to eat everything on your plate
- Soup fills you up and helps you feel full for longer
- Eat foods that you like, but be sensible! Avoid saturated fats. Reduce refined carbohydrates such as white bread, sugar, white flour. Cut down on salt
- Keep meals simple. Having too many varieties of food on the plate will encourage you to try everything, and to eat more than you need
- Make sure to have a varied diet with plenty of fruits and vegetables, to avoid nutritional deficiencies

EATING OUT

- Take a packed lunch to work, or prepare a tasty picnic for that day trip, instead of eating out or buying 'fast food'
- At the restaurant, order from the menu rather than having the 'All You Can Eat' buffet
- Order a starter as your main course
- Have one or two courses, rather than three
- Share a dessert with a friend
- Remember that alcoholic drinks are high in calories
- Read menu details, (and labels on shop-bought food!) – check for additives, salt, sugar and fats

It's hard to do it alone

Some people really appreciate the support of others when they are trying to lose weight. Local slimming groups can be found in many areas and are excellent if you need encouragement from others. If you don't want to go to such a group on your own, why not team up with a friend? Together you can attend a slimming club, join an exercise group, or even try a whole-food cookery course.

I weigh myself daily to see how much I've lost

Don't keep weighing yourself. Weight naturally fluctuates from week to week, sometimes from day to day, so you will not be getting a true picture by weighing yourself that often. You could get discouraged if you don't appear to have lost anything despite all your efforts, or if you are over the weight which you have decided is your target.

Weight loss can vary, even when you follow exactly the same meal plan each week, so don't be harsh on yourself or worry that you must have been 'over-eating'. Keep the weighing sessions to a minimum, perhaps once a week or fortnight. Each time do it at the same time of day, wearing similar clothing.

In any case, weight isn't necessarily an indication of body fat. Muscle weighs more than fat, so if you've been exercising you may actually gain weight, having gained muscle, even if you've lost a bit of fat. On the other hand, weight loss can be due to loss of fluids, perhaps because of dehydration or urination, so again it's not always a true measure of fat loss.

You don't need a set of scales to tell if you are trimmer. You can tell that by the way you feel, and how your clothes fit and hang on you. When you're eating a healthy diet, and perhaps getting some exercise, you will begin to feel better and will have more energy. This is more important than the amount of weight that has been lost. Constantly obsessing about the numbers is depressing and non-productive, and can keep you from enjoying your life and your food.

Is home-cooking worth the effort?

The big advantage of home-cooking is that you can control what goes into your dish, and it's also easier to control portion sizes. The food you cook yourself is likely to be fresher and higher in vitamins than a ready-prepared meal from the supermarket.

Ready-made dishes often contain high levels of fat, salt, sugar, preservatives, and inferior ingredients. Even so-called 'low-fat' foods do contain fat, and can include extra sugar and additives to compensate for lack of flavour. The calorie content of 'low-fat', 'reduced-fat' or 'extra-light' foods may actually be higher than a full-fat item, so always read the labels.

Home-cooking is not rocket science - simple, healthy and economic meals can be prepared with basic culinary skills. If necessary, get yourself a basic cookery book of simple, all-purpose recipes, or look for recipes on-line and in magazines. Perhaps surprisingly, excellent healthy recipes and advice on nutrition can also often be found in men's fitness & health magazines.

You might consider joining a local cookery class, especially if you prefer a bit of guidance. Suggestions for vegetarian meals can be obtained from the Vegetarian Society. See **Appendix II Contacts List**

Simple home-cooked meals can often be prepared in less time than it takes to go out and queue at the take-away shop or to wait for a pizza delivery. An additional advantage of home-cooking is that it involves exercise. Scrubbing, peeling, grating and chopping vegetables, kneading dough, beating eggs, washing-up, fetching pans from the cupboard – all these activities give exercise opportunities within your normal daily activities. See **Chapter 15 Exercise**

Sometimes I'm too tired or unwell to cook a proper meal

When you feel tired you are much less likely to prepare a good meal for yourself, and may be tempted by 'junk' food, opting for take-away or home delivery fast foods, with their high fat and sodium content. Therefore it's important to get enough sleep and rest, and if you need a nap in the afternoon, have one. (Don't forget to use your ventilator.)

Planning ahead can help for those times when you can't cook a meal from scratch because you are short of time, or too tired and under the weather. Keep a stock of useful tinned foods including fish, fruit, beans, chopped tomatoes, plus fresh foods such as eggs, fruit, onions and potatoes. Make good use of your freezer. When you are cooking soups, stews, rice, fishcakes etc. make double quantities, then chill and freeze the extra in individual portions.

When you need something easy, a very quick and simple meal can be made from a micro-waved potato with cottage cheese or tinned beans and tuna. Instead of potato, try a portion of cooked rice from the freezer, reheated in the microwave oven. For extra nutrition, serve with a small salad. Watercress, grated carrot and sliced tomato make a simple side dish.

Eggs are another good stand-by for those times you don't feel up to cooking or eating much. A simple boiled or scrambled egg, or perhaps a plain omelette, with whole-grain bread or toast, would be quick to prepare.

Cold food can be nutritious too. Try fresh fruit, canned fruit in natural juice, dried apricots, yoghurt, salad, tuna sandwich, cold cooked chicken, nuts, sunflower seeds.

If all else fails to tempt you a hot, milky drink will replenish fluids, give you energy, and keep you going, and would be a better idea than having nothing at all.

My problem is that I'm underweight

Being underweight could be a family trait. If your immediate family members are all thin, don't expect to alter your body's shape greatly, just accept that you are naturally slim. However, being underweight has associated health problems, so if you feel that your weight is too low it would be advisable to seek medical advice.

Too much exercise can be a contributing factor for low body weight. If you take a lot of exercise, or have a hectic lifestyle, your calorie intake may not be sufficient. You need enough to maintain your weight AND put some on, so do check this out. Another contributing factor can be smoking. Cigarettes suppress the appetite in some people – another good reason for giving them up! See **Chapter 14 Smoking**

I am following a special diet as I need to put weight on, so the more chocolate the better!

In some cases the Doctor may suggest a protein drink or food supplement to provide extra calories. Some supplements have sweet or savoury flavours and are simply added to water, to make a drink or shake. Others are tasteless and are added to hot drinks and soups. However, it is possible to have a balanced, nutritious diet and get extra calories without the use of food supplements, if your Doctor doesn't prescribe them.

While you are trying to *gain* weight you can have larger portions and higher calorie foods, but you should still aim to eat healthily and avoid saturated fats. Choose semi-skimmed milk, and lean protein such as tuna or skinless chicken.

Other good foods include dried fruits, bananas, seeds, honey, beans, lentils, cottage cheese, jacket potatoes, sweet potatoes and thick home-made soup. Choose foods which are dense, such as wholegrain bread and muesli. Lighter foods can fill you up but will provide fewer calories.

If you have a small appetite it may be beneficial for you to eat little and often, or have a milky drink between meals. Use semi-skimmed milk on cereals, for home-made fruit smoothies, and for hot bedtime drinks. Extra calories can be obtained by mixing skimmed milk powder into your milk. In addition to your meals you may like to have two or three snacks during the day, such as a piece of fruitcake with a drink, but limit snack foods containing saturated fats. Other snack ideas: celery with cream cheese or peanut butter, banana, yoghurt, avocado, cottage cheese with wholegrain or rye bread, nuts and dried fruit.

> *I am slightly underweight, but I do eat healthy food. My husband and I have an allotment so we have fresh vegetables, salads, and fruit all year long, which I love.*

With a small appetite it's possible that you don't eat sufficient fruit and vegetables, thereby missing out on essential vitamins and minerals. Make up for this by having fresh fruit juice, but don't over-do it as the acid in fruit juice can erode the enamel on your teeth.

Exercise can help you build muscle and increase your bodyweight. By all means get weight-gain tips from sports-related magazines and books, but do remember that their weight strategies are geared towards specific needs and goals. These magazines often assume that you are an athletic person who engages in regular competitive sports, but don't be tempted to overstep your personal abilities, because you could risk injuring yourself.

Also be aware that some articles are thinly veiled advertisements for food supplement companies, or gym equipment manufacturers. For unbiased advice consult your Physician. See also **Chapter 15 Exercise**.

In Brief

- Faddy diets do not work and can even damage your health
- Diet plans fail if you have to deny yourself your favourite foods
- You should never feel too hungry or too full
- Try our tips, and aim for a sustainable 'Diet for Life'
- Stop obsessing about calories and the number of pounds lost
- Home-cooking is great, and needn't be a chore
- Being underweight has its own problems
- Any sudden weight increase or loss should be investigated by your Physician
- Consult your Doctor for dietary advice if you're concerned about your weight, and get medical approval before starting on any extreme or restricted diet plan

CHAPTER 14

Smoking

Cigarette smoking is the greatest single cause of illness and premature death in the UK. The good news is: Stopping smoking can make a big difference to your health. It is never too late to stop smoking to greatly benefit your health.

Patient UK

Will it really make a difference if I give up smoking?

Inhaling other people's tobacco smoke (passive smoking) irritates the throat and lungs, and increases mucus production. It's not just a simple case of disliking the smell - the chemicals in tobacco smoke can seriously compromise your health and interfere with breathing. See **Chapter 11 Sensitivity to Indoor Pollution**.

Tobacco smoke irritates the tissues of the soft palate. This can cause swelling which narrows the air passageways, and can aggravate snoring, Sleep Apnoea and other respiratory problems.

If smoking is allowed in your household your machine's filters will need replacing more quickly. Check them every week.

If you, yourself, are a smoker, the effects of the tobacco smoke, and the associated risks to your health, are even greater. Although it may be hard, it would be better to quit the smoking habit before problems start to develop. However, those risks will start to reduce as soon as you stop smoking, and even if you've smoked for years it's never too late to give up,

What's the best way to give up?

First of all, think about your motivations for giving up. Whatever they are, it helps to always keep them in mind:

- Your medical condition is probably at the top of the list. It can be a strong wake-up call when you understand that tobacco smoke can badly affect respiratory conditions and could seriously damage your general health
- Then there are the effects of passive smoking on family members, especially children. By smoking, you damage not only your own health but that of your close family too
- You'll see financial benefits if you're no longer watching your money 'go up in smoke'
- Smoking affects your appearance and attractiveness. It discolours teeth, affects your skin and makes your breath unpleasant. You can get yellow staining on the fingers as a result of holding lighted cigarettes. The smell of stale tobacco smoke lingers on your clothes, on your hair and in your home
- Smoking dulls your taste buds and prevents you from fully enjoying your food
- There are potential fire hazards in the home caused by matches, lighters and smouldering cigarettes
- A strong habit like smoking can take over and control your life. Imagine having to leave a warm, comfortable office to stand out in the pouring rain, wind battering your face, desperately trying to light a sodden cigarette!

Giving up is easy for some people and they are able to do it alone. They have a strong resolve and are able to stop immediately. For others, however, it is not so easy, and they will need some assistance. Nicotine is an addictive drug and giving up can be a struggle for many people. Everyone is different, and what works for you may not work for someone else.

Some people go 'cold turkey'. They immediately dispose of all their tobacco, cigarettes and smoking supplies, so that they cannot be tempted in their own home. Others find they do better by gradually cutting down.

I just couldn't shake off my chesty cough and eventually consulted my GP. He told me I would not improve while I continued to smoke, and warned me of possible further, and more serious, complications. It really shook me up, and when I got home I threw away all my cigarettes.

How can I kick the habit?

'Habit' does often play a part in a continuing addiction. Many people are accustomed to lighting up in certain circumstances, such as after a meal, while reading the newspaper, or when enjoying a cup of coffee. If you have such a trigger-point, try changing your routine to break the habit. Replace the after-dinner coffee with a drink of water or juice. Instead of remaining at the dining table, get up and do something else – start the washing-up, phone a friend, check your emails, feed the birds in the garden – whatever works for you.

A potential slipping point could be when you're out enjoying a meal with friends. Even when you tell people you have given up smoking, you still may be offered a cigarette when others are lighting up, and that after-dinner habit could kick in again. Being aware of this possible pitfall will help you to cope with the temptation of your old habit.

However, if you do succumb and accept a cigarette, don't despair or think you have failed. Yes, you've given in to temptation, but put it behind you, move on, and be determined that it won't happen again. Don't beat yourself up; one slip does not make you a failure. It's important to stay positive and focus on your smoke-free goal.

I need help to give up cigarettes

In the UK the National Health Service offers a range of services to help you, including specialist advisers, postal/email programmes, local support groups and Nicotine Replacement Therapy (NRT). Various NRT products can be purchased without prescription - gum, sprays and patches. Ask at your Pharmacy. Helpful leaflets are usually available at Pharmacies and Doctors' surgeries. Your own Physician will be able to offer advice, and may prescribe medications.

For some, an unconventional incentive can be all the encouragement they need:

My mother-in-law made a wager that she'd give me a box of chocolates if I could last a month without smoking. She said I wouldn't be able to do it, but I did, and have never smoked again. By the way, the chocolates were delicious!

Hypnotherapy has helped many people to quit their addictive habits, and could be suitable for you. There are qualified therapists in most areas. You may prefer to purchase a self-hypnosis CD or DVD which you can use at home.

What else can I do to help myself?

Here are some suggestions which people have found useful:

- ◆ Rather than doing it alone, you might enlist the help of a friend or relative who is also trying to give up smoking. You can support, help and encourage each other through the process
- ◆ Look for helpful advice on the internet and check the NHS website. See whether your local library has any self-help books on the subject
- ◆ Try the 5 minute rule: When you feel like a cigarette, tell yourself that you'll have one in 5 minutes time. Go and get involved with doing something - a chore, a hobby, a phone call - to distract your mind from the urge to smoke. Hopefully it will be much longer than five minutes before you remember about the cigarette! Do the same thing whenever you feel the craving. It will help you achieve longer and longer intervals between cigarettes.
- ◆ Use lots of water, both inside and out. The aim is to rid your body of the nicotine as quickly as possible, to reduce your desire for the drug

  - Drinking plenty of water will help flush the nicotine out of your system, and will also give your mouth something to do instead of puffing on a cigarette. Reaching for a glass of water instead of that cigarette will help break the smoking habit, and it has no calories!
  - Keep your teeth clean to brush away any traces of nicotine from your mouth.

- Take frequent showers or baths to wash away nicotine from your body and hair: give your skin an invigorating rub to remove any nicotine which has been eliminated through the pores

- A warm bath or shower can ease tension and help you to relax if you're feeling the stress of withdrawal symptoms

- Baths and showers have another benefit – while you're in there, you're prevented from smoking as you can't light up a wet cigarette!

Will I put on weight if I stop smoking?

Cigarettes can suppress the appetite, and some people worry they will gain weight if they give up smoking. Also, without that cigarette they feel strange with nothing in the mouth, and they may replace it with candy, chewing gum or chocolate. Nicotine chewing-gum or sugar-free gum could help, or you might like to nibble on pieces of fresh fruit and vegetables. Try carrot sticks, apple and celery. Remember that too much candy can damage your teeth and lead to tooth decay.

> *By gradually cutting down on cigarettes I've managed to give up smoking completely, and it's amazing how good my food tastes now. It's like my taste buds have woken up! But I do try to resist the temptation to over-eat, especially the non-healthy stuff like cheesecake and chips.*

When you stop smoking you'll probably find that your senses of taste and smell improve. The food you eat seems to taste so much better, and this can encourage over-indulgence.

While being overweight has its own health implications, it is nevertheless important to persevere with giving up the tobacco. If you begin to snack too much, or crave sugary things, look for healthier options such as sugar-free gum, fresh fruit or a piece of wholegrain toast with low-fat spread. Or try the carrot sticks again! See **Chapter 13 Diet & Nutrition**.

In Brief

- It's never too late to give up smoking
- Find a method which suits you
- Ask a friend to give up with you, if you need extra support
- Use plenty of water – inside and out
- Watch your weight – you may be tempted to overeat when your taste buds recover and food tastes so good again
- Help is available: look for advice on-line etc
- Your Doctor can help you, or could refer you to a Stop Smoking Clinic

CHAPTER 15

Exercise

Physical activity is one of the most effective ways of positively influencing our health.

Age UK

Keeping active can contribute to improvements in your general and respiratory health, as can following good dietary habits and cutting out smoking. Regular exercise helps improve your stamina. It speeds metabolism and strengthens heart and lungs, while increasing physical endurance and muscle tone. It builds bone density, reduces the risk of osteoporosis and contributes to a healthy sleeping pattern, although you should not exercise too close to bedtime, as it may actually cause problems with sleeping.

Healthy activities and exercise are important. They improve fitness and contribute to a longer, healthier and more independent life. They can be a great help in maintaining a healthy body weight and reducing flab, so long as you don't copy this example:

I had a good workout session at the Gym. Then I went home and had supper in bed – biscuits and cheese, pork pie, scotch eggs and after-dinner mint chocolates!

At this point, are you thinking that you could skip this chapter? After-all, you're not planning to jog, can't do push-ups and aren't interested in all those other exertions which are associated with a serious work-out. If so, please let me emphasise that

EXERCISE **does** *NOT* **mean you have to go to the gym!**

In this chapter you will find suggestions for low-intensity exercises suitable for all abilities. Many of these can be done at home on your own. There is also advice for those who do wish to engage in the more active exercise options.

My breathing problems make exercise difficult – I'm not able to take part in strenuous activities. What kind of exercise could I possibly do?

The British Lung Foundation advises:

The reality is that we are surrounded by opportunities to be active in our daily lives. All it takes is a different perspective on the activities we already do.

It is not necessary to book yourself in for expensive sessions at a Health & Fitness Centre. Your daily life gives you many opportunities to be active, and your normal day-to-day activities all involve some form of exercise - preparing and cooking food, washing the dishes, walking the dog, ironing, knitting, housework, gardening, going for a good 'push' in your wheelchair, or strolling round the supermarket, even if you need to lean on your shopping cart.

I have learned to pace myself, and to rest when I need to. In nice weather I take a walk around the local lake. It has benches all the way round so if I need to stop for a rest it's not a problem.

Your own Physician may be able to arrange an appointment with a Physiotherapist who can help you put together a simple exercise routine suitable for your needs and abilities.

Sports Clubs and Leisure Centres often offer adult keep-fit classes, including sessions for those who are less able-bodied. Local support organisations such as Breathe Easy (organised by the British Lung Foundation) may be able to put you in touch with seated/wheelchair exercise groups (or 'chairobics') in your area. Other ideas for gentle exercise, suitable for doing at home or on your own, can be found later in this chapter. It is wise to seek medical advice before embarking on new or challenging physical activities, even those you do at home.

At the Gym – For the more active person

Some people are able to manage the more active forms of exercise. However, before embarking on any vigorous exercise regimen you should check with your Doctor, to make sure that what you are planning is suitable for you.

Once you have been given the go-ahead from your Doctor, you can look for someone to guide you in the higher intensity forms of exercise. Before you start working out with a gym instructor or a fitness trainer it is important to make sure that they are aware of any medical conditions you have, how those conditions affect you and what medications or treatments you are receiving. For example, some exercise routines include pulse monitoring. This may not be a reliable measure for you, if your usual pulse rate is faster than what is considered to be 'normal' in an able-bodied person. Your trainer needs to know this.

When taking out membership of a Gym or Health & Fitness Centre, you can make enquiries to check whether their instructors have received specialised training for dealing with disabled clients.

Remember that whatever form of exercise you do, you should start small and gradually build up.

People often think that exercise doesn't do you any good unless it hurts. Professional athletes may well follow this philosophy in order to reach the high standards which their sport requires. They are very fit people whose bodies can take the stresses and strains of high-level training. In their dedication to achieving their goals, they are prepared to accept physical damage. The aim of sports professionals or athletes is to be the best in their field.

For the rest of us, however, the objectives of exercise are to improve our health and to help us stay independent, and for us pain is a warning sign. Ignore it and you may damage yourself. Pain or discomfort tells you that you should take a break, or stop. If the exercise is hurting, then you should consult a qualified trainer for guidance and instruction on the correct way to perform the moves.

Always remember that some medications can mask pain. If you have been prescribed analgesic medication you may miss out on the painful feelings which act as warning signs, and therefore you could run the risk of getting hurt without even noticing.

To avoid injury always allow time for a warm-up before exercise. Do something light, such as gentle stretches. Shake your limbs out or do a few basic movements without using weights. During the exercise routine stay focused on what you are doing. If you let your mind wander you may not immediately notice tiredness or strain, and could put yourself at risk of avoidable damage. Don't rush what you're doing, and don't overdo it. You may think that an extra 20 or 30 minutes exercise must be beneficial, but it could put you at risk of injury. Towards the end of the session gradually wind-down the pace, rather than stop suddenly.

When you're feeling tired or under the weather, if you have a cough, or didn't sleep well the previous night, don't do anything strenuous. It's far better to take a day or two off than to risk further sickness or problems.

Muscle cramps and spasms during exercise may be caused by nutritional deficiencies, so stick to a varied, healthy diet, and ensure you keep yourself hydrated during the session. Do take a sensible view of your exercise, and stay within your limits. After all, your aim is to stay well and independent, rather than to become as fit as a professional athlete.

Won't I get fat if I stop exercising?

Contrary to the common myth, muscles will not turn to fat if you have to cut back on your exercise. You will, however, put weight on if you continue taking in the same amount of calories once you have reduced your energy output.

Think about a body-builder who performs regular exercises, and follows a special dietary regimen, designed to make the muscles of his body conspicuous for competitions. If he is not preparing for a competition he will cut down on his exercise regimen AND his special diet. He will go back to a more 'normal' pattern of eating while he is not in training. In the same way, to prevent weight gain, cut back on your food intake when you cut back on your physical activity.

Exercising would quickly bore me

Exercise doesn't have to be painful or boring. You need to find an enjoyable activity, within your own capabilities. Doing something you dislike quickly leads to boredom, and you won't stick at it. If you can take up more than one form of exercise the variety will help prevent you from getting bored.

See what is on offer in your own area; perhaps join a local class or group. Look for adverts at Sports Centres, Gym Clubs, Health Food Stores, Adult Education Centres, and in local newspapers.

Exercise ideas, including sitting exercises

Here are some exercise suggestions. Several of the following ideas can be used at home. You might find it helps to exercise to music.

Resistance Bands These resemble large, strong rubber bands which you can pull against, for a variety of exercises involving arms, legs and upper body. They are not expensive, are widely available and come in several strengths from light to heavy. You can use them whilst in a sitting position to work on your upper body and arms, so they are ideal for wheelchair users.

Weights – (Also known as Resistance Training) Weights can be improvised by using canned food, plastic bottles filled with water or sand, large smooth pebbles, alabaster eggs etc. Routines can be put together to suit wheelchair users.

If you outgrow these weights – if you find the exercise becomes too easy – perform the same exercises slower, tensing your muscles as you work them (but don't try to tense them as hard as you can!). Doing this, and imagining the weight to be heavier than it actually is, produces the same effects as the real weight, but without the dangers. During the run-up to their competitions bodybuilders use the same principle to pump up their muscles before going on stage.

Traditional P.T. Exercises (Also known as Callisthenics) Push-ups, sit-ups, knee-bends etc. require no equipment and can work wonders. Movements should be adapted to suit your abilities or medical condition. Gentle warm-up exercises are always important. It's advisable to check that you are doing the movements correctly, to avoid possible injury. Get some personal advice from an expert or find a good instruction book.

Don't be tempted to over-do it, you may injure yourself. There is no point in comparing your personal exercise achievements with those of other people. Everyone is different and will find some things easier than others - you are not in competition with each other. We each have our limitations and the standard we reach will differ from person to person.

I have short arms and a short body, so I find it easier to do more push-ups than my friend who has long arms. He, on the other hand, seems to be built for sit-ups, which I find more challenging.

Ignore the cliché of muscular athletes rattling off hundreds of their callisthenics at breakneck speed. For everyday fitness and strength, slow controlled repetition is the best plan. Stop when you feel pleasantly tired, NOT when you're gasping for breath or straining for that last rep. The purpose of exercise is to make you fitter, not to wear you out. Throughout his life Charles Atlas, fitness icon of the 1930s, performed his callisthenics in the above controlled manner, and taught it in his 'Dynamic Tension' course, which could be modified to suit age and ability.

Dancing is an excellent exercise which not only helps keep you fit, but also offers a great opportunity to socialise and make new friends. Don't feel you have to sign up for a passionate Rumba or spicy Salsa class, or compete with the Break-Dancers. Local dance classes often offer a good selection of dance styles, suitable for all abilities, and there may be regular Tea-Dances which you could attend. You don't have to join in every single dance, but can sit out whenever you need to. Some styles of dance are adaptable for wheelchair users. If you are a Country Music fan line-dancing will spin your spurs, and you won't need to find a dance partner!

Yoga Don't be discouraged by images of skinny men wrapping their bodies into pretzel shapes. Yoga is a complete discipline that encompasses breathing exercises, meditation techniques, and a wide variety of poses that help to relieve muscle tightness, and improve flexibility and circulation.

Tai Chi may appeal to you. It is a form of 'meditation in motion' using stylised movements, (cast out any ideas of flying kicks or breaking boards). There are several styles of Tai Chi but these are mainly variations on a theme. You learn a 'form' – a sort of dance with non-combative martial arts moves – where you grapple with imaginary opponents using slow, graceful sequences of movements. It need not be strenuous but may require some mental effort to master.

There are self-defence aspects to Tai Chi, but unless you are willing to devote your life to it, this part needn't concern you. This non-competitive art does not require a partner, and you can learn the basics from DVDs or books (available from booksellers or Martial Arts suppliers).

Pilates Invented by Joseph Pilates, this system involves specially designed exercises that improve muscle tone and flexibility through the use of muscle contractions. These are not gruelling, and are easily adapted to differing abilities.

Alexander Technique improves posture and reduces body stresses. Popular with singers, musicians and actors, it has a wide following. The technique is taught on a one-to-one basis, so you will need to pay for a tutor.

More ideas for activities. These can often be done by wheelchair users.
>   **Darts**
>   **Carpet Bowls**
>   **Fishing**
>   **Horse Riding**
>   **Wheelchair Basketball**
>   **Wheelchair/Armchair Exercises / Chairobics**
>   **Sailing**
>   **Swimming**

Singing Though not strictly an 'exercise', it is worth noting that some people with Sleep Apnoea and other lung conditions have derived benefit from singing. Regular singing and vocal exercises may help to improve breathing and strengthen the diaphragm, as well as contributing to a sense of accomplishment and enhanced self-esteem. Wendy Guevara (vocal coach and professional singer) says that she has seen improvement in the lung capacity of students with respiratory conditions. Her student Abigail explains:

> *I've been affected by asthma since I was a baby, and recently a bad virus brought on effects such as laryngospasm (closing up of the throat). Because of this I have been undergoing treatment. I have also taken up singing which has helped immensely with my breathing, as breathing techniques are so crucial to singing.*
> *With Wendy, my vocal coach, I have been focusing on breathing exercises which have worked my lungs. I have learned to breathe from my diaphragm and to take in deeper breaths, rather than the small shallow breaths I was taking before. This has not only improved my breathing, but also my vocals which were damaged by the virus. I am able to speak and sing much louder now*

and feel there has been a great improvement on my breathing.

I'd like to go swimming

Swimming is an excellent exercise, and many people feel the benefit of a regular swim. The buoyancy provided by water reduces the stress placed on your joints and muscles, and therefore this kind of exercise is less likely to cause damage. There are, however, some potential difficulties for those with lung conditions and restricted breathing.

> *The Doctor thought that swimming would be good exercise for me, as I have Scoliosis, so I started going to the 'Swimming for the Disabled' group at my local pool. Unfortunately I have restricted lungs and just couldn't co-ordinate my breathing with the swimming strokes. I kept swallowing water, which made my breathing worse, and I got exhausted.*

Chest deformities or weak breathing muscles may mean a reduced lung capacity, with difficulty in taking deep breaths. This will have an impact on the buoyancy of your body in the water, and you may find it hard to stay afloat without constant kicking or swimming strokes. This can lead quickly to exhaustion. If you have to struggle to keep your head out the water it will put a strain on your neck and back muscles. Try using a buoyancy or flotation aid, and do not swim out of your depth.

When it's an effort to stay afloat, and your face keeps getting submerged, there is a danger of water inhalation. Water can find its way into your lungs, and this further reduces your lung capacity and decreases your buoyancy. It could also occur if you are pushed under the surface by other pool users, whether by accident or intentionally in play.

People with respiratory problems may have a more rapid rate of breathing, and therefore find it hard to hold a breath long enough for the duration of a swimming stroke. They need to breathe in before their head is clear of the water. This again means there is a danger of swallowing water, and water inhalation may occur. If this happens to you, it may be preferable to swim on your back doing the backstroke, but take care to watch out for other people in the pool, so you can avoid colliding with them.

If the water is cold its low temperature could affect you much quicker than it affects other swimmers. As your body temperature falls you'll require more oxygen to keep warm, so your breaths will become more rapid, making it even harder to stay afloat. Never jump into cold water, but ease yourself into the pool gently. As soon as you begin to feel shivery get out of the water and warm yourself up.

Some local sports facilities hold swimming classes for people with disabilities. Such classes are often held in pools in which the water is warmer than for the usual public sessions. Warm water will help ease your muscles and allow you a greater range of movements, as well as preventing you from getting chilled.

Exposure to chlorine in the water might affect you, especially if you have an increased sensitivity to chemicals, so ensure that the pool you use is well ventilated, and use swimming goggles to protect your eyes. When the weather is warm enough, why not enjoy a swim in an outdoor pool?

I like the water but can't manage to swim

Even if you can't swim, you can still enjoy the fun of the water by taking part in pool exercises or an aqua aerobics class. These are suitable for many medical conditions and disabilities, including arthritis and fibromyalgia, and are an efficient way to burn off calories. You can do water exercise by yourself too.

Simply walking up and down in the pool can be enjoyable and will be beneficial – the water should be up to your armpits and, just as when you're swimming, it will give support and reduce the stress on your body. There's less strain than when doing similar exercise on land, and you can adjust the exercise movements to your own needs and abilities.

In Brief

- ◆ Exercise does not only mean going for a work-out in the gym
- ◆ Daily activities provide many opportunities for exercise
- ◆ Muscle doesn't turn to fat if you have to reduce your exercise
- ◆ Choose a form of exercise which appeals to you, to avoid boredom
- ◆ Some exercises and sports can be performed sitting down
- ◆ Choose something within your own capabilities, to avoid injury

- ◆ Don't try to keep up with someone who is fitter than you. Keep within your own limits, and pace yourself
- ◆ Swimming is a good form of exercise, but may be more difficult for those with restricted breathing
- ◆ Check with your Doctor before starting on your exercise regimen

Part 5
PRESENT DAY

Twenty years ago, when I was first introduced to my NIV Ventilator, I thought that normal life for me was at an end. The prospect of depending on a machine seemed very scary, especially as it involved having a mask over my face.

Despite my fears, I soon learned to deal with my new circumstances. Although I had been critically ill, the machine brought my condition under control and after a period of recovery I realised that life really was worth living again.

My motto is:

"The machine is your friend, not your enemy. Look after it and it will look after you".

Marion M Mason

APPENDICES

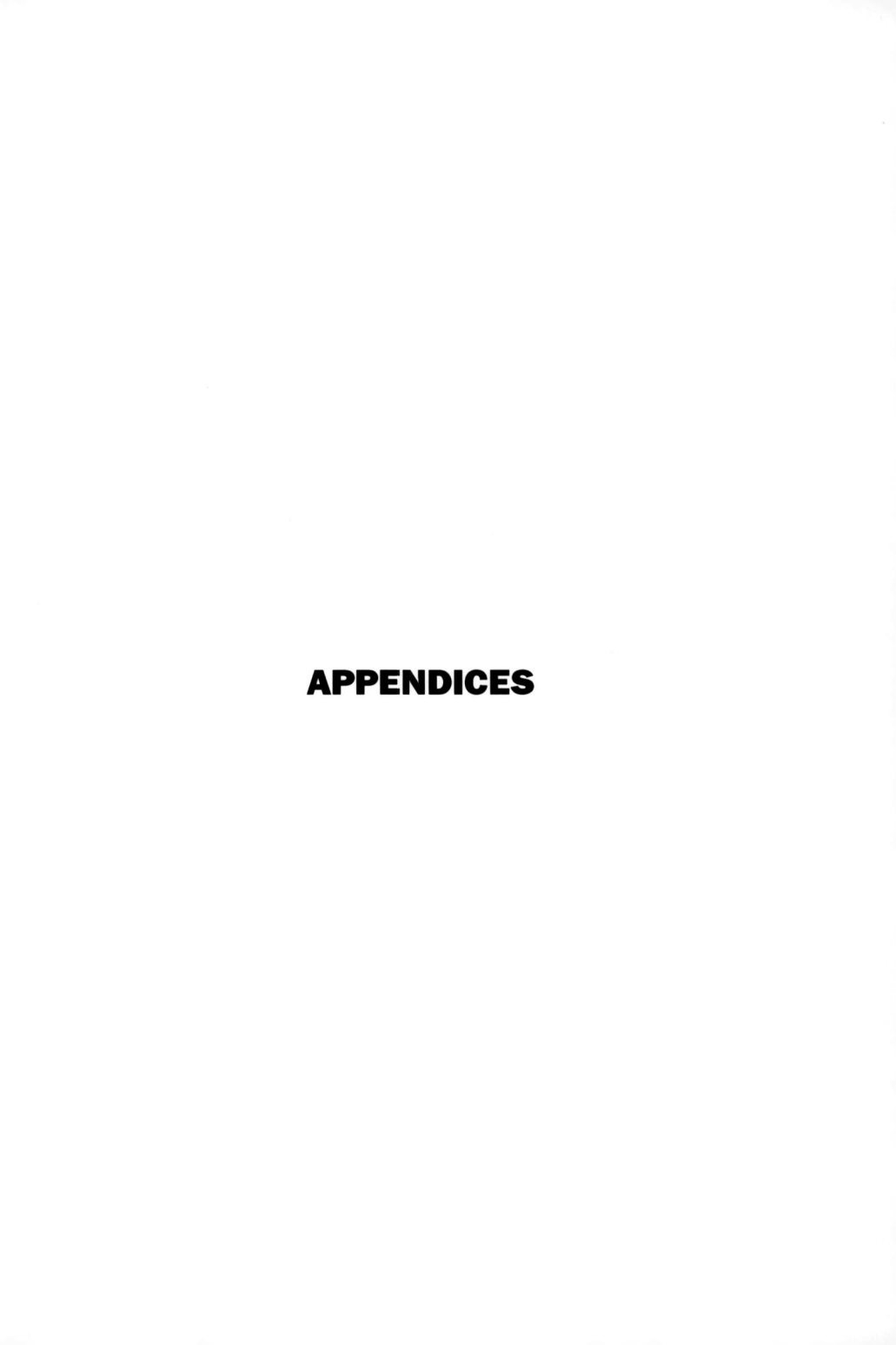

APPENDIX I

GLOSSARY OF TERMS & ACRONYMS

AEROPHAGIA
A condition when air passes into the oesophagus instead of the airway, filling the stomach and digestive tract, and causing distension

ARROW METHOD
Steve Mason's self-help technique for coping with negative emotions

BIPAP / BiPAP
Bi-level Positive Airways Pressure

CBT
Cognitive Behavioural Therapy
A psychotherapeutic approach that aims to solve problems concerning emotions, mood, anxiety etc.

CPAP
Continuous Positive Airways Pressure

CUIRASS
A rigid airtight body shell made of fibreglass or similar material. It encloses the patient's chest and trunk as he lies on his back. It is connected to a pump which delivers air into the shell under negative pressure

HUMIDIFIER
A piece of equipment sometimes used with CPAP or Ventilator. It provides heated humidification to reduce dryness of nose, mouth and throat

I.C.E
'In Case of Emergency'. Used on cell phone memory to indicate which number to call in the event of an emergency

IRON LUNG
A negative pressure tank consisting of a chamber which encloses the whole of the patient up to the neck

MECHANICAL RESPIRATORY SUPPORT
See NIV

MONNAL D
A portable but bulky positive pressure ventilator, superseded by smaller machines such as the Nippy

NIPPV
Non-invasive Positive Pressure Ventilation
NIPPY
Commonly used name for NIPPV ventilator
NIV
Non-Invasive Ventilation or Mechanical Respiratory Support
OSA
Obstructive Sleep Apnoea, usually the result of blockage or obstruction in the upper airway passages
OXIMETRY TEST
Measurement of blood oxygen levels
POLYSOMNOGRAPHY
A Sleep Study Test using electrode sensors on the head, and movement sensor bands around the chest.
SCOLIOSIS
Curvature of the spine.
Associated chest deformities can lead to ventilatory problems.
SLEEP APNOEA / SLEEP APNEA
Episodes of obstructed breathing while sleeping:
TIPPING-UP
Postural drainage of the airways using gravity
TRACHEOSTOMY
A surgical procedure in which an opening is made in the front of the windpipe (trachea)
UPPP
Uvulo-Palato-Pharyngo-Plasty
Surgical removal of the uvula & other soft fleshy parts of the throat
VPAP
Variable/bi-level Positive Airway Pressure

APPENDIX II

CONTACTS LIST

BOOKS
Picture Book for children:
A Monkey, a Mouse and a CPAP Machine
Contact: www.asiliveandbreathe.co.uk

BENEFITS ADVICE
ADVICE GUIDE
On-line advice & information on benefits, employment, housing etc
www.adviceguide.org.uk
BENEFITS ENQUIRY LINE (B.E.L.)
Tel: 0800 88 2200
CITIZENS ADVICE BUREAU
www.citizensadvice.org.uk

CARERS: SUPPORT ASSOCIATIONS & ORGANISATIONS
DIRECT GOV
Information for people with disabilities and their carers, including government services and information.
www.direct.gov.uk

CARERS UK
Information and advice for carers, on-line forums
UK	www.carersuk.org
Scotland	www.carersscotland.org
Wales	www.carerswales.org
N. Ireland	www.carersni.org

CROSSROADS
Information and support for carers
U.K.	www.crossroads.org.uk
Scotland	www.crossroads-scotland.co.uk
N.Ireland	www.crossroadscare.co.uk

EMERGENCY INFORMATION

MEDICAL TAGS
Tel: 0121 233 7455
www.medicaltags.co.uk

LIONS CLUB (Message in a Bottle)
www.lions.org.uk

MEDIC ALERT
Tel: 0800 581 420
www.medicalert.org.uk

SOS TALISMAN
www.medical-bracelets.co.uk

EMPLOYMENT

ACCESS TO WORK CONTACT CENTRES
Financial help for Employers & Disabled Employees
www.direct.gov.uk

ADVICE GUIDE
On-line advice & information on benefits, employment, housing etc
www.adviceguide.org.uk

EQUIPMENT & PRODUCT SUPPLIES

CPAP & NIV EQUIPMENT / ACCESSORIES etc

EU-PAP UK
www.eu-pap.co.uk
Tel: 0844-504-9999

CPAP Europe
www.CPAP-Europe.com
Tel: 0844-504-9999

CPAP Station (US)
www.cpapstation.com

Hope 2 Sleep
www.hope2sleep.co.uk
Tel: 0800 002 9711

FITNESS AND EXERCISE

AGE UK
Factsheets on exercise & healthy eating
www.ageuk.org.uk

NATIONAL INSTITUTE OF AGING
Exercise advice for older or less able people, including excellent illustrations for exercises you can do at home, both sitting and standing.
www.nia.nih.gov

WHEELCHAIR EXERCISES
www.thewheelchairsite.com/exercise/

FOOD & NUTRITION

AGE UK
Factsheets on exercise & healthy eating
www.ageuk.org.uk

BRITISH NUTRITION FOUNDATION
www.nutrition.org.uk

EAT WELL
Food Standards Agency:
www.eatwell.gov.uk

VEGETARIAN SOCIETY
www.vegsoc.org

FORUMS

CPAP & SLEEP APNOEA FORUMS:

www.cpap.co.uk

www.cpaptalk.com

www.hope2sleepguide.co.uk

www.talkaboutsleep.com

THE WHEEL LIFE   For wheelchair users
www.thewheellife.com

FRIENDSHIP, PEN PALS, DATING, RELATIONSHIP ADVICE

OUTSIDERS
Club for people who feel isolated by social or physical disability
Tel: 0207 354 8291
www.outsiders.org.uk
Email: info@outsiders.org.uk   for Club queries
         sexdis@outsiders.org.uk   for sexual problems
(See the website for Sex & Disability Helpline details)

MEDICAL CONDITIONS:
SUPPORT ASSOCIATIONS & ORGANISATIONS

ABLEIZE
UK Disability and Health Directory
www.ableize.com

ALLERGY ADVICE
www.allergyuk.org

AMERICAN LUNG ASSOCIATION
www.lungusa.org

ASTHMA
www.asthma.org.uk

AUSTRALIAN LUNG FOUNDATION
www.lungfoundation.org.au

BREATHE EASY GROUPS
see British Lung Foundation

BRITISH HEART FOUNDATION
Heart Matters Helpline: 0300-330-3311
www.bhf.org.uk

BRITISH LUNG FOUNDATION
Helpline: Tel: 08458-50-50-20
www.lunguk.org

BRITISH POLIO ORGANISATION
www.britishpolio.org.uk

BRITISH SNORING & SLEEP APNOEA ASSOCIATION
Tel: 01737-245638
www.britishsnoring.co.uk

CANCER RESEARCH
Tel: 020 7121 6699
www.cancerresearchuk.org

N.H.S. DIRECT
Tel: 0845 4647   24hours/7days
www.nhsdirect.nhs.uk

POLIO ASSOCIATION
www.polioassociation.org

THE SCOLIOSIS ASSOCIATION UK (SAUK)
Office: Tel: 0208 964 5343
Helpline: Tel: 0208 964 1166
www.sauk.org.uk

SLEEP APNOEA TRUST
www.sleep-apnoea-trust.org

SMOKING

N.H.S. STOP SMOKING SERVICES
Helpline: Tel: 0800 169 0 169
www.givingupsmoking.co.uk

TRAVEL & HOLIDAYS

CARE IN THE COUNTRYSIDE
Accessible holiday accommodation
www.careinthecountryside.net

FLYING WITH DISABILITY
Travel Advice
www.flying-with-disability.org

TRAVEL INSURANCE for people with medical conditions

ALL CLEAR TRAVEL
www.allcleartravel.co.uk

FREE SPIRIT
www.free-spirit.com

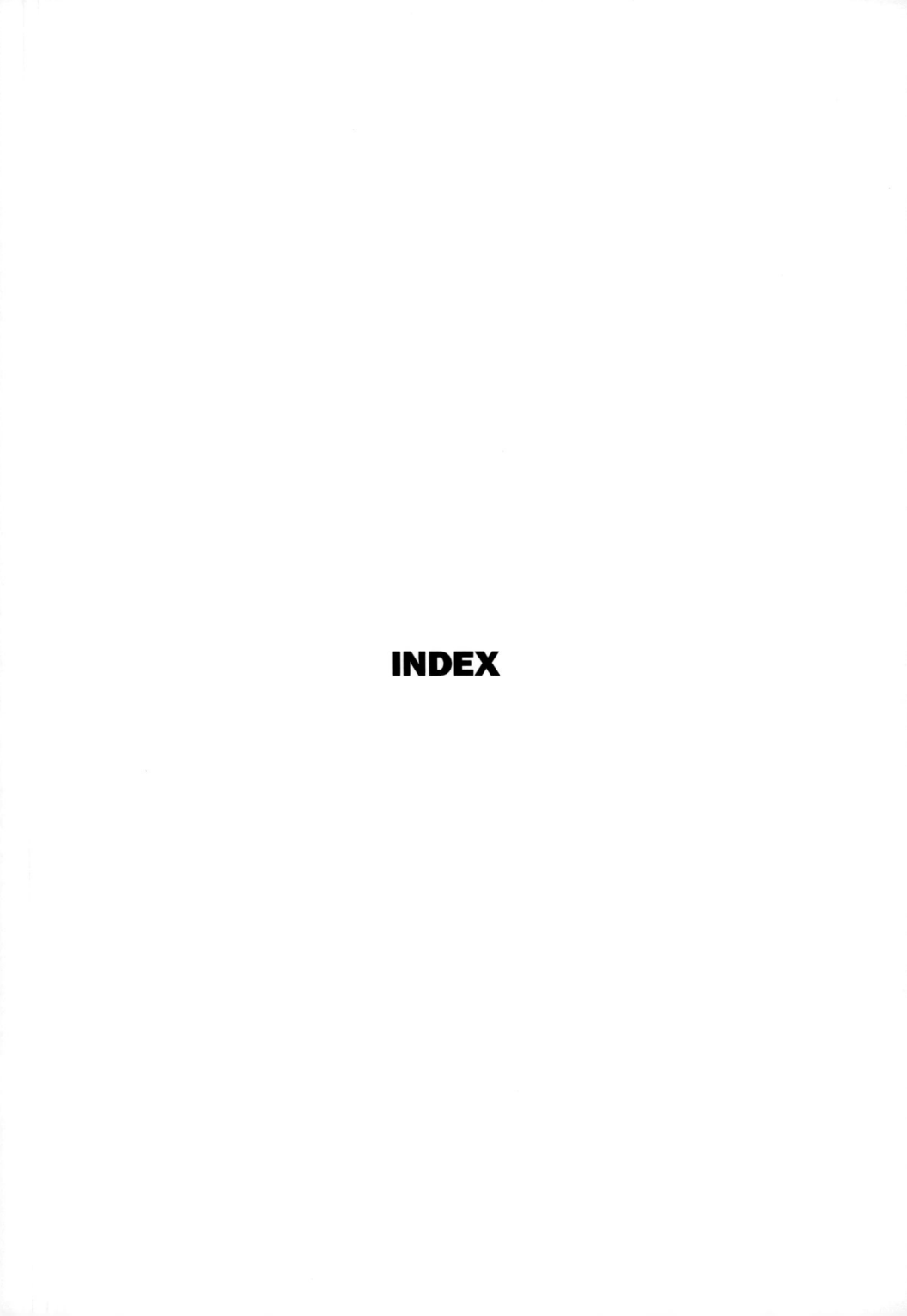

INDEX

INDEX

A
Advice and support   71-72, 75-76
Air leaks   See Mask
Alcohol, effects of   49-50
Allergies
        allergic reaction to mask   42
        sensitivity to household products   54, 111-113
Altitude, effect of changes   58-59

B
Beard   See Facial hair
Bed   See Comfort in bed
BIPAP   7, 9
Bloating   49
Blood gases/oxygen levels   8, 10, 11, 12, 45, 58

C
Children, reaction to the machine   73-74
Chinstrap   23, 32-33
        Photo page   99
Comfort in bed   29-34,
        Photos pages   96 & 99
Continuous positive airway pressure   8
        See also CPAP
CPAP   7, 8
        Photo page   96
CPAP Pillow   30
        Photo page   96
Cuirass   6
Cold nose   19, 34
Congestion, nose & chest   47-49

D
Diet and food
        breakfast   126

celebrity diets   124
diet for life - tips   127-128
extreme diets   124-125
home cooking   129-131
weighing yourself   129

E
Emergency health information   117-120
    Photos page   100
Emotions
    anxiety & negative emotions   101-107
making adjustments   68-70
    self esteem   67-68
Equipment
    faults   19-20
    filters   19, 20-21, 114, 135,
      Photos pages 94 & 95
    maintenance   19-23
    noise   85-87
Exercise
    at home   145
    benefits of exercise   141
    breathing problems & exercise   142, 148-149
    gym   142-144
    swimming   148

F
Facial hair   31, 37-38
Filters   19, 20-21, 114, 135
    Photos pages 94 & 95
Flight assessment test   59
Food   See Diet

H
Hose
    cleaning   22
    condensation in hose (rain-out)   18-19
    getting tangled in the hose   31-32

Hose-lift   18, 31-32, 42
    Photo page   99
Humidifier   18-19, 33

I
Indoor pollution   111-115
Iron lung   6
    Photos page   93
Lung capacity, restricted   9, 148

M
Mask
    air leaks   28-30
    allergic reaction to mask   42
    cleaning   21-22, 39
    damage to face   See Skin care
    dislodged by pillow   29-30
    pressure marks   34, 38
    straps   23, 27-28, 34
    types of mask   8, 26-27
        Photos pages   96, 98 & 99
Mechanical ventilation   5-7, 9
Monnal D   6, 7, 85
Moustache   See Facial hair
Mouth
    keeping mouth closed during sleep   32-33,
        Photo page 99
    secretions   32-33

N
Negative pressure chamber   6
NIV What is NIV?   5-7
NIPPY   7, 9
    Photos pages   94 & 95
NIPPV   9
Noise of equipment   28, 85-87

Nose
> blocked   47-49
> gets cold   19, 34
> soreness   33, 38, 42

O

OSA, obstructive sleep apnoea/apnea   7-9
Oximeter   10-11
Oximetry   10
Oxygen levels in blood   See Blood

P

Pillows, CPAP pillow   29-30
> Photo page 96

Polysomnography   11-12
Positive airway pressure   6-7
Power cuts   35-36
Pressure marks on face   See Mask

R

Rain-out   18-19
Relationships
> attractiveness   82-83, 88-90
> intimacy   87
> new partners   83-85
> noise of equipment   28, 85-87
> sleeping apart   87

S

Scoliosis   9, 148
Sensitivity to household products   54, 111-113
Skin care
> cleansing   38-39
> for men   37-38
> pressure marks   34, 38
> redness 40-41
> skin care products   38-41
> soreness   38-42

INDEX

171

       sun damage   40
       sun protection   40, 58
       vitamins   42-43
Sleep
       deprivation   8
       laboratory   11-12
       sleep apnoea / apnea   7-9
sleep study   10-12,
       Photos page 97
Smoking, effects on health   114, 135
Snoring   7-9, 10, 82, 86, 88, 90
Straps   23, 27-28, 34

T

Teeth, pain   30
Throat, soreness   18, 33
Travel
       air travel   59
       altitude changes   58-59
       doctor's advice   59, 60-61
       flight assessment test   59
       insurance   59-60
       taking oxygen supplies onto airplane   59, 61
       taking prescribed drugs with you abroad   60-61
       transporting your equipment   18, 61

By the same authors

A Monkey, a Mouse and a CPAP Machine
(Early Reader / Bed-time story for small children)

For more information visit our website
www.asiliveandbreathe.co.uk